Communications in Computer and Information Science 1773

Rationale

The CCIS series is devoted to the publication of proceedings of computer science conferences. Its aim is to efficiently disseminate original research results in informatics in printed and electronic form. While the focus is on publication of peer-reviewed full papers presenting mature work, inclusion of reviewed short papers reporting on work in progress is welcome, too. Besides globally relevant meetings with internationally representative program committees guaranteeing a strict peer-reviewing and paper selection process, conferences run by societies or of high regional or national relevance are also considered for publication.

Topics

The topical scope of CCIS spans the entire spectrum of informatics ranging from foundational topics in the theory of computing to information and communications science and technology and a broad variety of interdisciplinary application fields.

Information for Volume Editors and Authors

Publication in CCIS is free of charge. No royalties are paid, however, we offer registered conference participants temporary free access to the online version of the conference proceedings on SpringerLink (http://link.springer.com) by means of an http referrer from the conference website and/or a number of complimentary printed copies, as specified in the official acceptance email of the event.

CCIS proceedings can be published in time for distribution at conferences or as post-proceedings, and delivered in the form of printed books and/or electronically as USBs and/or e-content licenses for accessing proceedings at SpringerLink. Furthermore, CCIS proceedings are included in the CCIS electronic book series hosted in the SpringerLink digital library at http://link.springer.com/bookseries/7899. Conferences publishing in CCIS are allowed to use Online Conference Service (OCS) for managing the whole proceedings lifecycle (from submission and reviewing to preparing for publication) free of charge.

Publication process

The language of publication is exclusively English. Authors publishing in CCIS have to sign the Springer CCIS copyright transfer form, however, they are free to use their material published in CCIS for substantially changed, more elaborate subsequent publications elsewhere. For the preparation of the camera-ready papers/files, authors have to strictly adhere to the Springer CCIS Authors' Instructions and are strongly encouraged to use the CCIS LaTeX style files or templates.

Abstracting/Indexing

CCIS is abstracted/indexed in DBLP, Google Scholar, EI-Compendex, Mathematical Reviews, SCImago, Scopus. CCIS volumes are also submitted for the inclusion in ISI Proceedings.

How to start

To start the evaluation of your proposal for inclusion in the CCIS series, please send an e-mail to ccis@springer.com.

Buzhou Tang · Qingcai Chen · Hongfei Lin ·
Fei Wu · Lei Liu · Tianyong Hao ·
Yanshan Wang · Haitian Wang · Jianbo Lei ·
Zuofeng Li · Hui Zong
Editors

Health Information Processing

Evaluation Track Papers

8th China Conference, CHIP 2022
Hangzhou, China, October 21–23, 2022
Revised Selected Papers

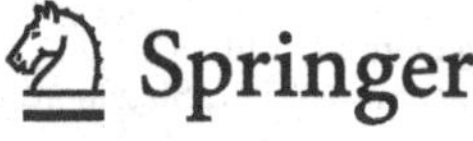

Editors
Buzhou Tang
Harbin Institute of Technology
Shenzhen, China

Qingcai Chen
Harbin Institute of Technology
Shenzhen, China

Hongfei Lin
Dalian University of Technology
Dalian, China

Fei Wu
Zhejiang University
Hangzhou, Zhejiang, China

Lei Liu
Fudan University
Shanghai, China

Tianyong Hao
South China Normal University
Guangzhou, China

Yanshan Wang
University of Pittsburgh
Pittsburgh, PA, USA

Haitian Wang
The Chinese University of Hong Kong
Shatin, New Territories, Hong Kong

Jianbo Lei
Medical Informatics Center of Peking University
Beijing, China

Zuofeng Li
Takeda Co. Ltd.
Shanghai, China

Hui Zong
West China Hospital
Chengdu, China

ISSN 1865-0929 ISSN 1865-0937 (electronic)
Communications in Computer and Information Science
ISBN 978-981-99-4825-3 ISBN 978-981-99-4826-0 (eBook)
https://doi.org/10.1007/978-981-99-4826-0

This Springer imprint is published by the registered company Springer Nature Singapore Pte Ltd.
The registered company address is: 152 Beach Road, #21-01/04 Gateway East, Singapore 189721, Singapore

Preface

Health information processing and applications is an essential field in data-driven life health and clinical medicine and it has been highly active in recent decades. The China Health Information Processing Conference (CHIP) is an annual conference held by the Medical Health and Biological Information Processing Committee of the Chinese Information Processing Society (CIPS) of China, with the theme of "Information processing technology helps to explore the mysteries of life, improve the quality of health and improve the level of medical treatment". CHIP is one of the leading conferences in the field of health information processing in China and turned into an international event in 2022. It is also an important platform for researchers and practitioners from academia, business and government departments around the world to share ideas and further promote research and applications in this field. CHIP 2022 was organized by the Harbin Institute of Technology (Shenzhen) and the proceedings were published by Springer. Due to the effects of COVID-19, the CHIP 2022 conference was held online, whereby people could freely connect to live broadcasts of keynote speeches and presentations.

The CHIP 2022 evaluation competition released 5 shared tasks with the theme of Medical Multimodal Information Extraction, including Text Mining for Gene-Disease Association Semantics, Medical Causal Entity and Relation Extraction, Medical Decision Tree Extraction from Unstructured Text, OCR of Electronic Medical Documents, and Clinical Diagnosis Coding. A total of 228 teams from more than 100 institutions participated in the shared tasks, of which 15 high-ranking teams submitted the algorithm papers. The organizer of the shared tasks also submitted 5 overview papers. The 20 papers were selected for publication in this volume after peer review and rigorous revision.

The authors of each paper in this volume reported the novel results of their proposed algorithms. The volume cannot cover all aspects of Medical Health and Biological Information Processing but may still inspire insightful thoughts for the readers. We hope that more secrets of Medical Multimodal Information Extraction will be unveiled, and that academics will drive more practical developments and solutions.

May 2023

Buzhou Tang
Qingcai Chen
Hongfei Lin
Fei Wu
Lei Liu
Tianyong Hao
Yanshan Wang
Haitian Wang
Jianbo Lei
Zuofeng Li
Hui Zong

Organization

Honorary Chairs

Hua Xu	UTHealth, USA
Qingcai Chen	Harbin Institute of Technology (Shenzhen), China

General Co-chairs

Hongfei Lin	Dalian University of Technology, China
Fei Wu	Zhejiang University, China
Lei Liu	Fudan University, China

Program Co-chairs

Buzhou Tang	Harbin Institute of Technology (Shenzhen) & Pengcheng Laboratory, China
Tianyong Hao	South China Normal University, China
Yanshan Wang	University of Pittsburgh, USA
Maggie Haitian	WangChinese University of Hong Kong, China

Young Scientists Forum Co-chairs

Zhengxing Huang	Zhejiang University, China
Yonghui Wu	University of Florida, USA

Publication Co-chairs

Fengfeng Zhou	Jilin University, China
Yongjun Zhu	Yonsei University, South Korea

Evaluation Co-chairs

Jianbo Lei	Medical Informatics Center of Peking University, China
Zuofeng Li	Takeda Co. Ltd., China

Publicity Co-chairs

Siwei Yu	Guizhou Medical University, China
Lishuang Li	Dalian University of Technology, China

Sponsor Co-chairs

Jun Yan	Yidu Cloud (Beijing) Technology Co., Ltd., China
Buzhou Tang	Harbin Institute of Technology (Shenzhen) and Pengcheng Laboratory, China

Web Chair

Kunli Zhang	Zhengzhou University, China

Program Committee

Wenping Guo	Taizhou University, China
Hongmin Cai	South China University of Technology, China
Chao Che	Dalian University, China
Mosha Chen	Alibaba, China
Qingcai Chen	Harbin Institute of Technology (Shenzhen), China
Xi Chen	Tencent Technology Co., Ltd., China
Yang Chen	Yidu Cloud (Beijing) Technology Co., Ltd., China
Zhumin Chen	Shandong University, China
Ming Cheng	Zhengzhou University, China
Ruoyao Ding	Guangdong University of Foreign Studies, China
Bin Dong	Ricoh Software Research Center (Beijing) Co., Ltd., China
Guohong Fu	Soochow University, China
Yan Gao	Central South University, China
Tianyong Hao	South China Normal University, China

Shizhu He	Institute of Automation, Chinese Academy of Sciences, China
Zengyou He	Dalian University of Technology, China
Na Hong	Digital China Medical Technology Co., Ltd., China
Li Hou	Institute of Medical Information, Chinese Academy of Medical Sciences, China
Yong Hu	Jinan University, China
Baotian Hu	Harbin University of Technology (Shenzhen), China
Guimin Huang	Guilin University of Electronic Science and Technology, China
Zhenghang Huang	Zhejiang University, China
Zhiwei Huang	Southwest Medical University, China
Bo Jin	Dalian University of Technology, China
Xiaoyu Kang	Southwest Medical University, China
Jianbo Lei	Peking University, China
Haomin Li	Children's Hospital of Zhejiang University Medical College, China
Jiao Li	Institute of Medical Information, Chinese Academy of Medical Sciences, China
Jinghua Li	Chinese Academy of Traditional Chinese Medicine, China
Lishuang Li	Dalian University of Technology, China
Linfeng Li	Yidu Cloud (Beijing) Technology Co., Ltd., China
Ru Li	Shanxi University, China
Runzhi Li	Zhengzhou University, China
Shasha Li	National University of Defense Technology, China
Xing Li	Beijing Shenzhengyao Technology Co., Ltd., China
Xin Li	Zhongkang Physical Examination Technology Co., Ltd., China
Yuxi Li	Peking University First Hospital, China
Zuofeng Li	Takeda China, China
Xiangwen Liao	Fuzhou University, China
Hao Lin	University of Electronic Science and Technology, China
Hongfei Lin	Dalian University of Technology, China
Bangtao Liu	Southwest Medical University, China
Song Liu	Qilu University of Technology, China
Lei Liu	Fudan University, China
Shengping Liu	Unisound Co., Ltd., China

Xiaoming Liu	Zhongyuan University of Technology, China
Guan Luo	Institute of Automation, Chinese Academy of Sciences, China
Lingyun Luo	Nanhua University, China
Yamei Luo	Southwest Medical University, China
Hui Lv	Shanghai Jiao Tong University, China
Xudong Lv	Zhejiang University, China
Yao Meng	Lenovo Research Institute, China
Qingliang Miao	Suzhou Aispeech Information Technology Co., Ltd., China
Weihua Peng	Baidu Co., Ltd., China
Buyue Qian	Xi'an Jiaotong University, China
Longhua Qian	Suzhou University, China
Tong Ruan	East China University of Technology, China
Ying Shen	South China University of Technology, China
Xiaofeng Song	Nanjing University of Aeronautics and Astronautics, China
Chengjie Sun	Harbin University of Technology, China
Chuanji Tan	Alibaba Dharma Hall, China
Hongye Tan	Shanxi University, China
Jingyu Tan	Shenzhen Xinkaiyuan Information Technology Development Co., Ltd., China
Binhua Tang	Hehai University, China
Buzhou Tang	Harbin Institute of Technology (Shenzhen), China
Jintao Tang	National Defense University of the People's Liberation Army, China
Qian Tao	South China University of Technology, China
Fei Teng	Southwest Jiaotong University, China
Shengwei	Tian Xinjiang University, China
Dong Wang	Southern Medical University, China
Haitian Wang	Chinese University of Hong Kong, China
Haofen Wang	Tongji University, China
Xiaolei Wang	Hong Kong Institute of Sustainable Development Education, China
Haolin Wang	Chongqing Medical University, China
Yehan Wang	Unisound Intelligent Technology, China
Zhenyu Wang	South China Institute of Technology Software, China
Zhongmin Wang	Jiangsu Provincial People's Hospital, China
Leyi Wei	Shandong University, China
Heng Weng	Guangdong Hospital of Traditional Chinese Medicine, China

Gang Wu	Beijing Knowledge Atlas Technology Co., Ltd., China
Xian Wu	Tencent Technology (Beijing) Co., Ltd., China
Jingbo Xia	Huazhong Agricultural University, China
Lu Xiang	Institute of Automation, Chinese Academy of Sciences, China
Yang Xiang	Pengcheng Laboratory, China
Lei Xu	Shenzhen Polytechnic, China
Liang Xu	Ping An Technology (Shenzhen) Co., Ltd., China
Yan Xu	Beihang University, China and Microsoft Asia Research Institute, China
Jun Yan	Yidu Cloud (Beijing) Technology Co., Ltd., China
Cheng Yang	Institute of Automation, Chinese Academy of Sciences, China
Hai Yang	East China University of Technology, China
Meijie Yang	Chongqing Medical University, China
Muyun Yang	Harbin University of Technology, China
Zhihao Yang	Dalian University of Technology, China
Hui Ye	Guangzhou University of Traditional Chinese Medicine, China
Dehui Yin	Southwest Medical University, China
Qing Yu	Xinjiang University, China
Liang Yu	Xi'an University of Electronic Science and Technology, China
Siwei Yu	Guizhou Provincial People's Hospital, China
Hongying Zan	Zhengzhou University, China
Hao Zhang	Jilin University, China
Kunli Zhang	Zhengzhou University, China
Weide Zhang	Zhongshan Hospital Affiliated to Fudan University, China
Xiaoyan Zhang	Tongji University, China
Yaoyun Zhang	Alibaba, China
Yijia Zhang	Dalian University of Technology, China
Yuanzhe Zhang	Institute of Automation, Chinese Academy of Sciences, China
Zhichang Zhang	Northwest Normal University, China
Qiuye Zhao	Beijing Big Data Research Institute, China
Sendong Zhao	Harbin Institute of Technology, China
Tiejun Zhao	Harbin Institute of Technology, China
Deyu Zhou	Southeast University, China
Fengfeng Zhou	Jilin University, China
Guangyou Zhou	Central China Normal University, China
Yi Zhou	Sun Yat-sen University, China

Contents

Medical Decision Tree Extraction from Unstructured Text

OCR of Electronic Medical Document

Clinical Diagnostic Coding

Text Mining for Gene-Disease Association Semantic

Text Mining Task for "Gene-Disease" Association Semantics in CHIP 2022

Sizhuo Ouyang, Xinzhi Yao, Yuxing Wang, Qianqian Peng, Zhihan He, and Jingbo Xia(✉)

Hubei Key Lab of Agricultural Bioinformatics, College of Informatics, Huazhong Agricultural University, Wuhan, Hubei, People's Republic of China
xjb@mail.hzau.edu.cn

Abstract. Gene-disease association plays a crucial role in healthcare knowledge discovery, and a large amount of valuable information is hidden in the literature. To alleviate this problem, we designed and organized the Gene-Disease Association Semantics (GDAS) track in CHIP2022, which aims to automatically extract the semantic association between the gene and disease from the literature. The GDAS track includes three progressive subtasks, gene-disease concept recognization, semantic role labeling, and gene-regulation-disease triplet extraction. Six teams participated in the track and submitted valid results, three of which showed promising performance in the GDAS track, we briefly present and summarize their methods. Finally, we discuss the potential value of the GDAS track to the healthcare and BioNLP communities, and explore the feasibility of further methods to facilitate the GDAS track.

Keywords: Named entity recognition · Semantic role labeling · Triplet extractionevgevee · Gene-disease association · Natural language processing

1 Introduction

China Health Information Processing (CHIP) Conference is an annual conference held by the Medical Health and Bioinformation Processing Committee of the Chinese Information Processing Society of China (CIPS). Adhering to the theme of "Using information processing technology to help explore the mystery of life, improve the quality of health and improve the level of medical treatment", the conference has held to eighth session. Health information processing is the core content in the field of life health and clinical medicine, which has been a wide concern for a long time. The eighth CHIP Conference focuses on "digital and intelligent medical health", gathering the country's top medical information processing scholars and medical experts. The purpose of the conference is to jointly discuss the trends and challenges of smart medical development, new methods of medical research, and new ways of artificial intelligence in medical applications [1].

B. Tang et al. (Eds.): CHIP 2022, CCIS 1773, pp. 3–13, 2023.
https://doi.org/10.1007/978-981-99-4826-0_1

To mine gene-disease association information useful for health care from biological literature, this paper initiates an evaluation track "Gene-Disease Association Semantic Mining Task" [2], focusing on entity information and semantic roles in massive literature. All the data in the evaluation task are collected from Active Gene Annotation Corpus (AGAC) [3], which marks entity types and relationships between entities. The annotation guidelines of AGAC are elaborated in [4]. Statistics on the annotation of the train set and test set refer to Wang et al. [5]. In addition to AGAC, some other biological corpora have focused on the relationship between mutations and diseases. The GENIA corpus [6] is a semantically annotated corpus of biological literature with the core topic of medicine and its related fields. The annotated content mainly focuses on biological reactions related to human blood cell transcription factors. The CRAFT corpus [7] is a collection of journal articles on phenotypic ontological "annotation" evidence in mice, featuring a "multi-model" annotation task that focuses on genomic information. These corpora mainly focus on biological concepts and different biological reactions caused by their mutation information. Guided by biological concepts, they extend to the medical field and connect the interdisciplinary knowledge discovery of biology and medicine.

The AGAC has a wide range of applications, like predicting key genes of Alzheimer's disease (AD), extracting mutant genes, and the biological process, in which these genes are involved in regulation [8]. The obtained AD-related literature is filtered based on rules such as text correlation, then the filtered texts are annotated with AGAC. The results suggest that 325 mutations are extracted, and 822 pairs of positive/negative regulation-related mutation triples and their corresponding sentence evidence are obtained. These 325 mutations all carry clear semantic information of downstream biological processes caused by the mutation. The corresponding sentence evidence can prove the correctness of the extracted triplet information, indicating that AGAC has shown great potential in the exploration of key genes in the field of AD, as well as the ability of sustainable in-depth analysis. It can also be applied in the relocation of anti-epilepsy drugs [3]. These anti-epilepsy target drugs are not documented in the database but are supported by literature, which promotes drug reuse. A total of 281 gene-drug pairs, including 112 drugs and 28 genes, are obtained through PubMed. Additionally, "mutation" and "epilepsy" are used as keywords to filter and annotate the literature abstracts. The predictions are matched against entries in the DrugBank database. 112 drugs are recorded by 30 drugs in the database. Of the 10 newly predicted multi-target drugs that are not in the inventory, 6 are found to be associated with epilepsy and all are supported by the literature. In addition, it can also be used to mine the mutation logical chain in the literature related to COVID-19 [9]. Thus, it can predict which downstream biological phenomena will be affected by the mutation of the virus and whether the virus will be more likely to infect the host cells.

The AGAC is originally designed to address the problem of gene labeling with changes in central function. The definition of "functional change" derives from the focus on the loss of function and gain of function. The corpus is designed by Wang et al. [4], which contains 500 manually annotated abstracts collected from PubMed. The molecular objects, regulations, and semantic roles contained in AGAC are listed in Table 1. Nine molecular objects are Disease, Gene, Protein, Enzyme, Mutation, Interaction, Pathway, Molecular Physiological Activity (MPA), and Cellular Physiological Activity (CPA). And three types of regulation conceptual entities: Positive Regulation (PosReg), Negative Regulation (NegReg), and Regulation (Reg). In addition, AGAC also describes topic and causality through the two semantic roles of Theme and Cause.

Table 1. Annotation types identified in AGAC. (a) Entity types and labels. (b) Semantic role types.

(a)

Entity Types	Named Entities	Entity Label
Molecular objects	Gene	Gene
	Disease	Disease
	Protein	Protein
	Enzyme	Enzyme
	Mutation	Var
	Pathway	Pathway
	Cellular Physiological Activity	CPA
	Molecular Physiological Activity	MPA
	Interaction	Interaction
Regulations	Regulation	Reg
	Positive Regulation	PosReg
	Negative Regulation	NegReg

(b)

Relations	Semantic Roles	Relation Label
Between molecular objects	Theme	ThemeOf
Between molecular object and regulation	Cause	CauseOf

In this study, we introduced the overview of the task design, organization of GDAS track in CHIP 2022, provided the evaluation results of the task, and finally gave further discussion of the shared task in biomedical and healthcare knowledge discovery.

2 Materials and Methods

2.1 The Motivation of the GDAS Track

The motivation of the GDAS track is to solicit more natural language processing (NLP) methods and provide an evaluation of NLP engineering capabilities.

The GDAS track focuses knowledge discovery on the characteristic field of gene-disease associations through a series of common NLP community tasks, such as named entity recognition and relational extraction of semantic roles. AGAC has been successfully applied to LitCovid [10], the literature data set related to COVID-19, and launch the joint annotation corpus LitCovid-AGAC [9]. The annotation results of the corpus explore the AGAC annotation related to the novel coronavirus mutation. Its downstream mechanism and its mechanism confirmation, as shown in Fig. 1.

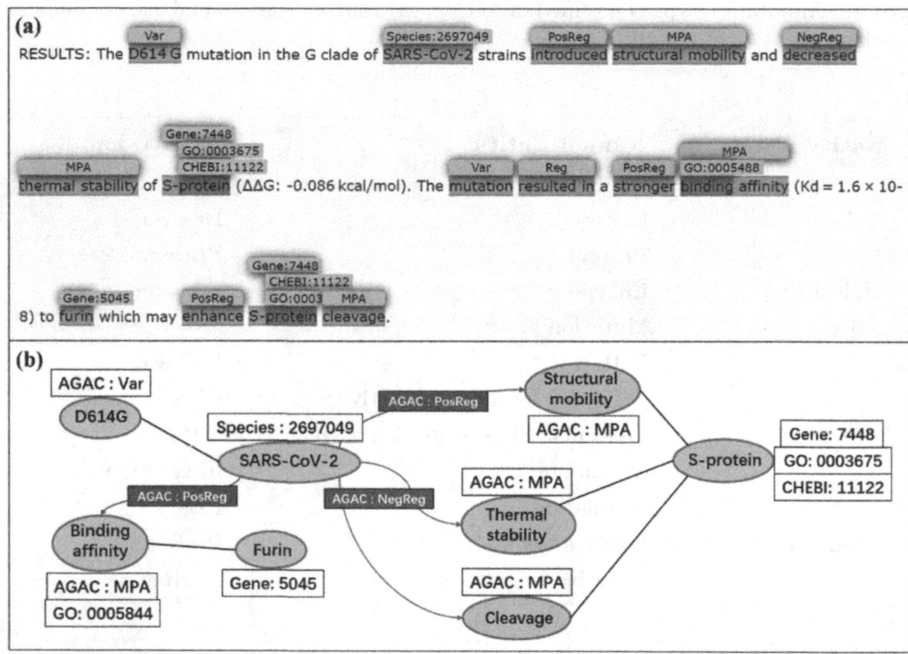

Fig. 1. AGAC labeling and mechanism illustration related to "Novel coronavirus mutation and its downstream mechanism".

The D614G mutation in the G branch of the SARS-CoV-2 strain resulted in the structural mobility of the S protein, thereby reducing its thermal stability. However, the mutation can enhance the binding affinity between furin protease and S protein, so that cleavage of S protein can be enhanced [11]. It can be seen that the latent logic chain and biological knowledge in the literature have the significance of in-depth exploration. The GDAS track can facilitate the discovery of customized knowledge literature for diseases similar to COVID-19 among other diseases. It also reflects that the GDAS track connects the interdisciplinary communication between biology and medicine.

2.2 GDAS Track Design

The JSON format is used for data in GDAS tasks. Figure 2 shows a specific JSON file that contains all the information for annotations. The content in each JSON file is

```
{"target": "http://pubannotation.org/xxxxxxxx",
"sourcedb": "PubMed",
"sourceid": "xxxxxxxx",
"text": "xxxxxx",
"denotations": [{"id": "xx", "span": {"begin": xx, "end": xx}, "obj":
    "xxx"}, {"id": "xx", xxxxxxx}, ...],
"relations": [{"id": "xx", "pred": "xxx", "subj": "xx", "obj": "xx"},
    {"id": "xx", xxxxxxx}, ...]}
```

"*target*" is the PubAnnotation link for each annotated text. "*sourcedb*" means the text source, all texts in AGAC are from PubMed. "*sourceid*" is the PMID of each text. "*denotations*" contains the annotation information in task 1, of which the "*id*" represents the unique identification of each annotated entity, the "*span*" represents the start and end positions of the entity and the "*obj*" is the label assigned to the entity. "*relations*" contains the semantic roles between two entities, the "*id*" represents the unique identification of each semantic role, the "*pred*" is the semantic role from "*subj*" to "*obj*".

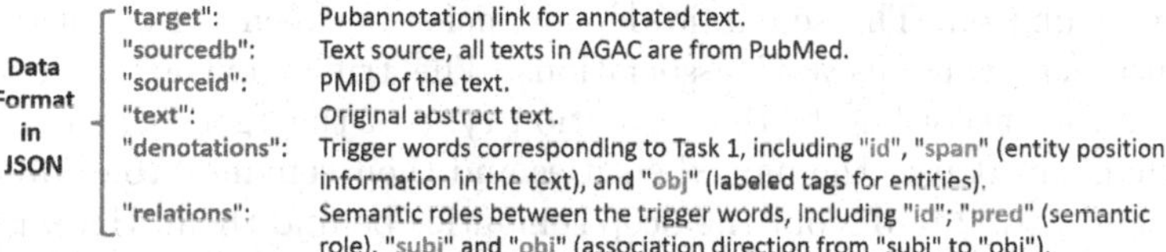

{"target": "http://pubannotation.org/docs/sourcedb/PubMed/sourceid/25805808", "sourcedb": "PubMed", "sourceid": "25805808", "text": "Loss-of-function de novo mutations play an important role in severe human neural tube defects.\nBACKGROUND: Neural tube defects (NTDs) are very common and severe birth defects that are caused by failure of neural tube closure and that have a complex aetiology. Anencephaly and spina bifida are severe NTDs that affect reproductive fitness and suggest a role for de novo mutations (DNMs) in their aetiology.\nMETHODS: We used whole-exome sequencing in 43 sporadic cases affected with myelomeningocele or anencephaly and their unaffected parents to identify DNMs in their exomes.\nRESULTS: We identified 42 coding DNMs in 25 cases, of which 6 were loss of function (LoF) showing a higher rate of LoF DNM in our cohort compared with control cohorts. Notably, we identified two protein-truncating DNMs in two independent cases in SHROOM3, previously associated with NTDs only in animal models. We have demonstrated a significant enrichment of LoF DNMs in this gene in NTDs compared with the gene specific DNM rate and to the DNM rate estimated from control cohorts. We also identified one nonsense DNM in PAX3 and two potentially causative missense DNMs in GRHL3 and PTPRS.\nCONCLUSIONS: Our study demonstrates an important role of LoF DNMs in the development of NTDs and strongly implicates SHROOM3 in its aetiology.", "project": "AGAC2_PubMed_2","denotations": [{ "id": "T8", "span": { "begin": 771, "end": 778 }, "obj": "Protein" }, { "id": "T7", "span": { "begin": 779, "end": 789 }, "obj": "NegReg" }, { "id": "T6", "span": { "begin": 790, "end": 794 }, "obj": "Var" }, { "id": "T9", "span": { "begin": 823, "end": 830 }, "obj": "Gene" }, { "id": "T10", "span": { "begin": 936, "end": 939 }, "obj": "NegReg" }, { "id": "T11", "span": { "begin": 940, "end": 944 }, "obj": "Var" }, { "id": "T12", "span": { "begin": 961, "end": 965 }, "obj": "Disease" }, { "id": "T3", "span": { "begin": 1224, "end": 1227 }, "obj": "NegReg" }, { "id": "T1", "span": { "begin": 1228, "end": 1232 }, "obj": "Var" }, { "id": "T2", "span": { "begin": 1255, "end": 1259 }, "obj": "Disease" }, { "id": "T5", "span": { "begin": 1284, "end": 1291 }, "obj": "Gene" }], "relations": [{ "id": "R1", "pred": "CauseOf", "subj": "T1", "obj": "T3" }, { "id": "R10", "pred": "ThemeOf", "subj": "T12", "obj": "T10" }, { "id": "R11", "pred": "ThemeOf", "subj": "T5", "obj": "T1" }, { "id": "R2", "pred": "ThemeOf", "subj": "T2", "obj": "T3" }, { "id": "R5", "pred": "CauseOf", "subj": "T6", "obj": "T7" }, { "id": "R6", "pred": "ThemeOf", "subj": "T8", "obj": "T7" }, { "id": "R7", "pred": "ThemeOf", "subj": "T9", "obj": "T6" }, { "id": "R8", "pred": "ThemeOf", "subj": "T9", "obj": "T11" }, { "id": "R9", "pred": "CauseOf", "subj": "T11", "obj": "T10" }]}

Fig. 2. Data example in JSON format

The GDAS track is divided into three sub-tasks in Fig. 3: trigger-named entity recognition, semantic role labeling, and triplet extraction of "Gene, Regulation type, Disease".

Twelve types of named entities will be identified in task 1, including nine molecular objects and three regulations. These have been defined in Table 1(a).

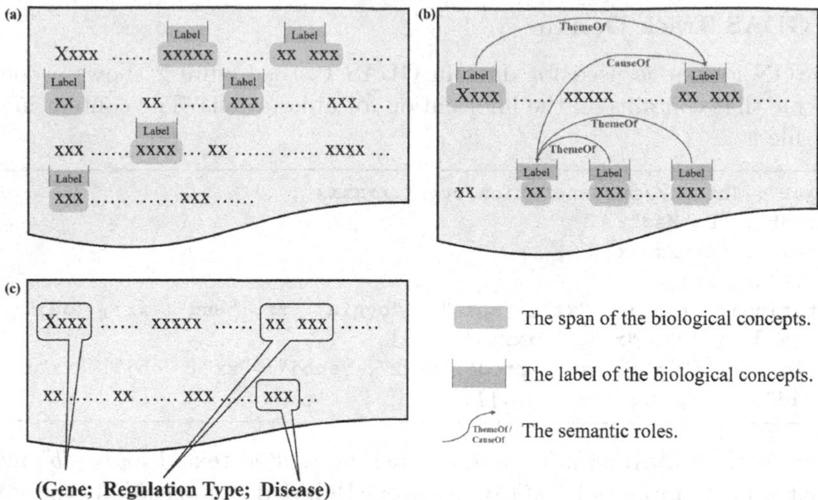

Fig. 3. The setting of the GDAS track tasks. (a) Task 1: trigger-named entity recognition. (b) Task 2: semantic role labeling. (c) Task3: triplet extraction of "Gene, Regulation type, Disease".

Based on this, semantic role labeling will annotate the "ThemeOf" relation between molecular objects and the "CauseOf" relation between molecular objects and regulation. The semantic dependencies between these entities are used to construct "gene-disease" associations. The triplet extraction extracts relevant semantics according to the regulation type of the "gene-disease" association mechanism. It uses the named entities and their semantic roles obtained from task 1 and task 2 to dig out the deep semantics behind them. Here, regulation types include four semantic descriptions of mutated genes: Loss Of Function (LOF), Gain Of Function (GOF), Regulation(REG), and Compound change of a function (COM). The GDAS track provides the results of the "Gene, Regulation Type, Disease" triad of 250 training texts. Of the three tasks, task 2 is based on task 1, and task 3 can be performed independently or based on the results of task 1 or task 2.

2.3 Evaluation Metrics

The results of the participating teams are evaluated through standard "Precision", "Recall", and "F1-score".

$$Precision = \frac{TP}{TP + FP}, \tag{1}$$

$$Recall = \frac{TP}{TP + FN}, \tag{2}$$

$$F1 - score = \frac{2 \times Precision \times Recall}{Precision + Recall}, \tag{3}$$

where TP is true positives, FP is false positives and FN is false negatives.

The evaluation tool "PubAnnotation Evaluator" from PubAnnotation is used for task 1 and task 2. And the parameter settings for strict span matching are considered. If task 2 is to judge whether the predicted relationship is true positive, it is necessary to correctly predict the two entities participating in the relationship and the type of relationship. For task 3, our organizer has provided a customized evaluation tool that uses the Macro-F1, precision and recall automatically generated from the Sklearn toolkit in Python.

2.4 The Task Organization of the GDAS Track

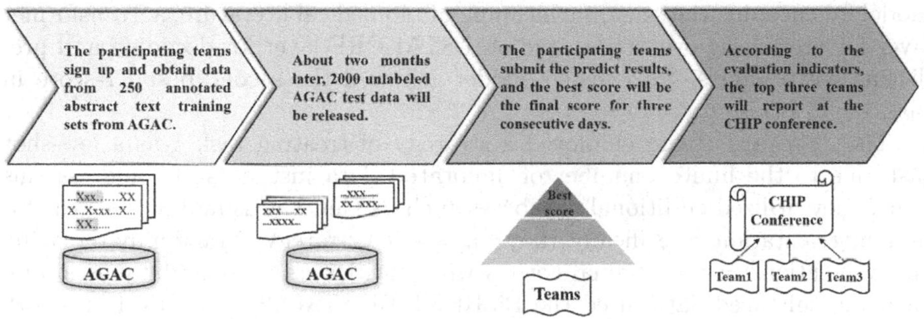

Fig. 4. The task organization of the GDAS track.

Figure 4 is the task organization of the GDAS track. Generally, teams interested in participating in the GDAS track should first register with our organizer and sign a commitment letter on data use and confidentiality. Then they would obtain 250 annotated abstract text and triplet extraction results from AGAC as the training set. In about two months' time, we will publish a total of 2000 texts without annotations as testing data from AGAC. We provide a three-day period for participating teams to submit predicted results and evaluate the results. The highest score of each team in these three days shall be taken as the final score of the team. The top three teams will be presented and reported at the CHIP conference.

3 Results

3.1 Overview of the Top Three Performing Teams

During the eighth CHIP Conference, this assessment task attracted nearly 20 teams from universities and enterprises to participate in the competition. Finally,

6 teams submitted valid competition results. The best results in task 1 and task 2 were from the "WinHealth" team of Weining Health Technology Co. The best result in task 3 is the "Forward" team from Beijing Jiaotong University.

Task 1. In task 1, "WinHealth" achieved the highest F1-score of 0.52, followed by "Deep Hide Blue" with an F1-score of 0.44, and "Forward" placed third, with an F1-score of 0.41.

The "WinHealth" team constructed an end-to-end model for joint learning of the three tasks by exploring potential semantic connections among them. They utilized a pre-trained BERT model, Global Pointer, and Partition Filter Network for learning textual embedding representations, joint feature learning, and informal interactions among multiple tasks, respectively. This team's model ultimately achieved the highest F1-score in task 1.

The "Deep Hide Blue" team utilized a stacked model architecture to handle the data features of the AGAC corpus. They employed a pre-trained BioBERT model for encoding the semantic meaning of biomedical literature, a Transformer layer for preventing overfitting, and an LSTM-CRF layer for decoding and predicting entity labels. This team's model achieved the second-best F1-score in task 1.

The "Forward" team employed a strategy of treating task 1 as a few-shot task due to the limited number of annotated data instances. To address this issue, they utilized additional databases such as GeneCards and MalaCards for data augmentation. Specifically, they employed a strategy of randomly replacing entity mentions in the original corpus with entities from these databases and, with the enhanced data, used the BioBERT-BiLSTM-CRF generic framework for biomedical entity recognition. This team achieved promising results in task 1.

Task 2. In task 2, "WinHealth" achieved the highest F1-score of 0.31, followed by "Forward" with an F1-score of 0.03.

The "WinHealth" team leveraged the recursive information from task 1 to enhance the performance of relationship extraction. Similar to task 1, the team used a pre-trained BERT model to learn relevant RE features.

The "Forward" team applied their previously established data argumentation strategy to task 2 and tested a variety of models for relation extraction. Ultimately, they achieved their best results using the TDEER model coupled with data augmentation.

Task 3. In task 3, "Forward" achieved the highest F1-score of 0.61, while "WinHealth" placed second with an F1-score of 0.24.

The "Forward" team employed their data argumentation strategy and TDEER model from task 2, which resulted in the best performance.

The "WinHealth" team used the explicit relationship inference obtained from task 2 predictions to enhance the performance of inferring potential gene-disease relationships. They utilized a shared feature that combines the features from the NER task in task 1 and the SRL task in task 2 for implicit relationship inference in task 3.

The precision, recall, and F1-score of all teams across the three tasks are summarized in Table 2. Of note, while "WinHealth" achieved better results than the baseline model in task 1, all teams performed worse than the baseline in task 2 and task 3, highlighting the need for more research on these more challenging tasks.

We can note that out of all six participating teams, only two teams participated in all three tasks at the same time, while the others only participated in task 1. We have analyzed the reasons for this as follows. On the one hand, The results show that even the best-performing teams had limited success in tasks 2 and 3, demonstrating the difficulty of semantic role extraction and moderated reasoning in the biomedical literature. Furthermore, the results show that achieving a high ranking in these tasks is heavily dependent on a good performance in task 1. The limited participation in task 2 and task 3 further highlights the need for continued research and innovation in these areas to advance biomedical natural language processing. Despite the challenges encountered in the competition, the variety of strategies and techniques employed by the teams demonstrates the potential and promise of the AGAC corpus and its application in biomedical research.

3.2 Results of All Participating Teams

Six teams participated in the track, of which all teams participated in task 1, and only "WinHealth" and "Forward" participated in task 2 and task 3. Table 2 shows the precision, recall, and F1-score of all teams, which are summarized as follows:

- Task 1 is the most basic but important task with most participants, in which "WinHealth" achieves the best precision of 0.55 and F1-score of 0.52; "Deep Hide Blue" achieves the best recall of 0.51.
- Task 2 and task 3 are more challenging than task 1 and therefore involve fewer participants. In task 2, "WinHealth" achieves the best precision of 0.32, recall of 0.31, and F1-score of 0.31. In task 3, "Forward" achieves the best precision of 0.77 and F1-score of 0.50; "Deep Hide Blue" achieves the best recall of 0.61.
- "WinHealth" achieves better results than baseline in task 1, but all teams do worse than baseline in task 2 and task 3, which leads us to hope that more researchers will focus on these two more challenging tasks.
- Considering the results of the three tasks, the ranking of the participating teams is shown in column "Team" in the table.

Table 2. Results of all participating teams.

	Task 1			Task 2			Task 3		
Team	Precision	Recall	F1-score	Precision	Recall	F1-score	Precision	Recall	F-Score
WinHealth	**0.55**	0.49	**0.52**	**0.32**	**0.31**	**0.31**	0.46	0.18	0.24
Forward	0.37	0.46	0.41	0.02	0.06	0.03	**0.77**	**0.50**	**0.61**
Deep Hide Blue	0.38	**0.51**	0.44	-	-	-	-	-	-
NLP small group	0.30	0.33	0.32	-	-	-	-	-	-
YLab	0.52	0.18	0.27	-	-	-	-	-	-
test001	0.01	0.01	0.01	-	-	-	-	-	-
Baseline*	0.50	0.51	0.50	0.84	0.82	0.83	0.72	0.59	0.65

-: The team did not attend the evaluation.
*: Baseline provided by the task organizer.

4 Discussion and Conclusion

The AGAC corpus and the GDAS track task have shown great potential for the biomedical natural language processing field. The text-mining track for "Gene-Disease" association semantics based on the AGAC corpus has significant application prospects and highlights the potential of the corpus.

Performances of attendant teams in GDAS track have shown the success of the-state-of-arts NLP schemes, some of which outperformed the Baseline. It is noteworthy that the AGAC guideline's judgment is whether a sentence carries sufficient semantic information to trigger a label. Each annotation result has analytical significance, inspiring applications of the corpus in customized and accurate knowledge mining for biomedical and healthcare semantic information. The evaluation encourages further development of customized corpus and conventional NLP methods toward corpus-based knowledge discovery setting.

Very recently, the rise of huge scale pre-trained language models, such as ChatGPT and GPT4, emerges and suggests promising application for various NLP tasks. The future discussion of applying huge scale pre-trained language model into the current knowledge discovery task is indispensable, and GDAS track is one of the case fallen in this scope. Huge scale language model opens up a new possibility for improving the performance in the GDAS track and scaling up corpus construction.

From a point view of fact, tasks like GDAS track heavily rely on manual annotation corpora of a small or medium sizes. In the meantime, the annotation logic in these corpora are usually delicate and complex, taking AGAC as an example. Therefore, the sophisticated knowledge design in corpus ensures the knowledge correctness, while the huge scale pre-trained models have demonstrated remarkable semantic understanding. These developments will undoubtedly further advance biomedical NLP overall progress and achieve more significant application prospects. With a high chance, the combination of both corpus-based NLP methods and huge scale pre-trained language model is a promising way leading to both abundant and accurate knowledge discovery.

Acknowledgements. The work is funded by the Fundamental Research Funds for the Central Universities (No. 2662021JC008, No. 2662022XXYJ001), and the Major Project of Hubei Hongshan Laboratory (No. 2022HSZD031).

References

1. Zong, H., Lei, J., Li, Z., et al.: Overview of technology evaluation dataset for medical multimodal information extraction. J. Med. Indform. **43**(12), 2–5+22 (2022)
2. Ouyang, S., Yao, X., Wang, Y., Peng, Q., He, Z., Xia, J.: An overview of the text mining task for "gene-disease" association semantics. J. Med. Indform. **43**(12), 6–9 (2022). (in Chinese)
3. Wang, Y., et al.: An active gene annotation corpus and its application on anti-epilepsy drug discovery. In: 2019 IEEE International Conference on Bioinformatics and Biomedicine (BIBM), pp. 512–519. IEEE (2019)
4. Wang, Y., et al.: Guideline design of an active gene annotation corpus for the purpose of drug repurposing. In: 2018 11th International Congress on Image and Signal Processing, BioMedical Engineering and Informatics (CISP-BMEI 2018), Oct 2018, Beijing (2018, accepted)
5. Wang, Y., Zhou, K., Gachloo, M., Xia, J.: An overview of the active gene annotation corpus and the BioNLP OST 2019 AGAC track tasks. In: Proceedings of the 5th Workshop on BioNLP Open Shared Tasks, pp. 62–71 (2019)
6. Kim, J.-D., Ohta, T., Tateisi, Y., Tsujii, J.: Genia corpus-a semantically annotated corpus for bio-textmining. Bioinformatics **19**(suppl_1), i180–i182 (2003)
7. Cohen, K.B., et al.: The colorado richly annotated full text (CRAFT) corpus: multi-model annotation in the biomedical domain. In: Ide, N., Pustejovsky, J. (eds.) Handbook of Linguistic Annotation, pp. 1379–1394. Springer, Dordrecht (2017). https://doi.org/10.1007/978-94-024-0881-2_53
8. Zhou, K., et al.: Bridging heterogeneous mutation data to enhance disease gene discovery. Brief. Bioinform. **22**(5), bbab079 (2021)
9. Ouyang, S., Wang, Y., Zhou, K., Xia, J. LitCovid-AGAC: cellular and molecular level annotation data set based on COVID-19. Genom. Inform. **19**(3) (2021)
10. Chen, Q., Allot, A., Zhiyong, L.: LitCovid: an open database of COVID-19 literature. Nucleic Acids Res. **49**(D1), D1534–D1540 (2021)
11. Mohammad, A., Alshawaf, E., Marafie, S.K., Abu-Farha, M., Abubaker, J., Al-Mulla, F.: Higher binding affinity of furin for SARS-CoV-2 spike (S) protein D614G mutant could be associated with higher SARS-CoV-2 infectivity. Int. J. Infect. Dis. **103**, 611–616 (2021)

Hierarchical Global Pointer Network: An Implicit Relation Inference Method for Gene-Disease Knowledge Discovery

Yiwen Jiang[1(✉)] and Wentao Xie[2]

[1] Winning Health Technology Group Co., Ltd., Shanghai, China
j_yw@winning.com.cn

[2] School of Methematics and Statistics, Beijing Institute of Technology, Beijing, China
xwt0016@bit.edu.cn

Abstract. The investigation of new associations between genes and diseases is a crucial knowledge extraction task for drug discovery. In this paper, we present a novel approach to gene-disease knowledge discovery in the 8th China Health Information Processing Conference (CHIP 2022) [31] Open Shared Task AGAC Track (http://www.cips-chip.org.cn/2022/eval1). Selective annotation and latent topic annotation are two major challenges in this task. To address these challenges, we propose a novel Hierarchical Global Pointer Network with propagation module to extract implicit relations that are inferred based on explicit relations. We are also the first one to design a unified end-to-end model which can achieve three AGAC tasks simultaneously and alleviate the problem of selective annotation. The experiment results show the method we proposed can achieve F1-scores of 52%, 31% and 30% for three tasks respectively.

Keywords: drug repurposing · gene-disease association · hierarchical global pointer network

1 Introduction

Drug repurposing, which refers to the identification of new uses for approved drugs beyond their original medical indications, is regarded as an alternative for novel drug discovery. Since marketed drugs have undergone sufficient clinical trials and are approved for safety and efficacy, investigating new associations between diseases and marketed drugs is more efficient than developing new drugs.

Finding novel disease-drug associations is the main work of drug repurposing. Generally, pathogenic genes or target genes are the hub to associate diseases and drugs. The active gene annotation corpus (AGAC) [13,14,22], which contains manually annotated abstracts collected from PubMed (a significant source of scientific knowledge discovery) [4] was created as a benchmark dataset for the objective of drug repurposing. AGAC was developed to capture function

B. Tang et al. (Eds.): CHIP 2022, CCIS 1773, pp. 14–28, 2023.
https://doi.org/10.1007/978-981-99-4826-0_2

changes of mutated genes i.e., loss of function (LOF) and gain of function (GOF), in biomedical text. It has been successfully exploited to predict Alzheimer's disease-related genes [30] or enhance the process of antiepileptic drug discovery [24]. Supposing that the information of LOF/GOF can be automatically extracted from loads of biomedical literature through Natural Language Processing (NLP) techniques, large scale prediction of drug candidates for diseases will be accomplished because the association between drugs and targeted genes were recorded in databases like DrugBank [27] or Therapeutic Target Database [11].

The design of AGAC is highly motivated by the experimentally supported LOF-agonist/GOF-antagonist hypothesis [25], which stated that a targeted antagonist/agonist is a candidate drug for a given disease resulted from a mutated gene with GOF or LOF. AGAC under the hypothesis consists of three tasks [23]: 1) trigger words Named Entity Recognition (NER), 2) thematic relation extraction, and 3) gene-disease triplet extraction. Task 1 involves twelve types of named entities, which are relevant to genetic variations and forthcoming phenotype changes. These entities can be categorized into bio-concepts, regulation types and other entities related to molecular or cellular levels. In Task 2, two thematic relation types, "Theme" and "Cause", are designed to interlink semantic dependency between AGAC entities. After mutation, a gene either loses or gains a function. Task 3 highlights a LOF/GOF-classified gene-disease association is expressed by a triplet as *(gene, type of function change, disease)*. Such triplet is the most straightforward form of knowledge piece to understand the related pathology and thus, apply the hypothesis for drug discovery. Although each of these AGAC tasks can be conducted independently, Task 2 might require the result of Task 1, and Task 3 might be benefited from the results of other 2 tasks semantically.

Selective annotation and latent topic annotation are two unique features introduced in AGAC guidelines [22]. Selective annotation means that not all named entities appearing in a sentence will be annotated. Only those sentences which clearly carry sufficient information about function changes e.g., specific gene, mutation and disease mentions, are annotated. This character stems from the real scenario of drug knowledge discovery and make the NER task of AGAC more complicated one compared to typical NER tasks. Relational information included in Task 2 and Task 3 might contribute to distinguishing whether a sentence should be annotated or not, since these relations prompt clues of function changes. In addition, the LOF/GOF context of a gene-disease association may not be expressed directly in the text, so the annotation of AGAC Task 3 may be regarded as a kind of latent topic annotation. This feature requires NLP models to fully understand the abstract and utilize the shallow semantic knowledge from Task 2, so as to infer the implicit gene-disease association.

In this paper, we consider Task 1 as standard medical NER task and regard both Task 2 and Task 3 as relation extraction (RE) tasks. We can also further subclassify Task 2 and Task 3 as explicit relation extraction (ERE) and implicit relation extraction (IRE) respectively. To conquer the aforementioned annotation challenges, we design an end-to-end joint model to simultaneously realize three AGAC tasks, facilitating the information sharing among multi-tasks.

Specifically, inspired by the Partition Filter Network (PFN) [28] that models balanced bi-directional interaction between NER and RE tasks, we modify this architecture to generate three task-specific features. The encoder with gate mechanism in PFN partitions each neuron into intra-task partitions and inter-task shared partition. Information valuable to both NER and RE tasks e.g., features related to function changes in AGAC, is stored in shared partition to improve the performance of selective annotation. In addition, we propose a novel Hierarchical Global Pointer Network (HGPN) with message-passing paradigm to infer implicit relations based on the first-extracted shallow semantic knowledge. Similar to Graph Attention Networks [19], a self-attention based propagation module is integrated into a token-pair linking unit to learn semantically enhanced representations which are part of the input to next hierarchy layer. In summary, our contributions include:

1. To our best knowledge, we are the first one to propose an end-to-end model that simultaneously achieves three AGAC tasks through the encoder of Partition Filter Network, ensuring proper interaction among multi-tasks to solve the selective annotation problem.
2. Following the feature of latent topic annotation, we propose a novel Hierarchical Global Pointer Network with propagation module for implicit relation reasoning.
3. We conduct experiments on AGAC test dataset, and the experimental results demonstrate the validity of our method. The overall performance won the first place in the 8th China Health Information Processing Conference (CHIP 2022) AGAC track.

2 Related Work

The AGAC was first studied in BioNLP Open Shared Task 2019 [23]. Li et al. [10] integrated pre-trained language models into a pipeline method for Task 1 and Task 2. Liu et al. [12] proposed a joint model based on a multi-task learning framework for joint inference on NER and thematic relation extraction. However, selective annotation remains an unresolved problem in previous work. Their approaches extract features for different tasks in the same predefined order, under which relation signals about function changes cannot affect NER features to label selectively. For Task 3, Thillaisundaram et al. [17] extended BERT with minimal task-specific architecture to encode and classify the LOF/GOF-relation of mention pairs. Latent topic annotation has not been explored, as none of thematic relations in Task 2 were jointly learned for implicit relation inference. Moreover, none of the previous works jointly model the whole three tasks and fully exploit the correlation among different tasks to alleviate the problem of selective annotation and latent topic annotation.

At present, the main discriminative approaches for joint entity and relation extraction can be broadly classified into sequence labeling [7,26,29] and table-filling based approach [3,20,21]. Sequence labeling involves assigning one or more labels to each token in a sentence to locate the starting and ending positions of entities and relations. Table-filling based approach is to enumerate all spans within a sentence, creating a table and classifying each element in it. Although these methods can effectively extract entities and relations jointly, there is few research on dividing relations into explicit and implicit types, as well as developing a model that can extract both types of relations in one step, leveraging explicit relations for better implicit relation inference.

3 Problem Formulation

AGAC consists of three tasks: NER, ERE and IRE. Formally, given an input sentence $s = \{w_1, w_2, \ldots, w_L\}$ with L tokens, w_i denotes the i-th token in sequence s. NER task aims to extract all entity mentions $\langle w_s, e, w_e\rangle \in S$ with selective annotation, where w_s and w_e represent the start and end token of an entity typed $e \in E$. E represents the set of pre-defined AGAC entity types e.g., Gene and Disease. The set of entities recognized in Task 1 is denoted by S. For RE tasks, including both ERE and IRE, the goal is to identify all relations between entities in S. Each relational triple is denoted by $\langle w_i, w_j, r, w_m, w_n\rangle \in T$, where $\langle w_i, w_j\rangle \in S$ and $\langle w_m, w_n\rangle \in S$ indicate the subject and object entities respectively in relation r. In Task 2, there are two thematic relation types $r \in R_e$, where $R_e = \{\text{“}ThemeOf\text{”}, \text{“}CauseOf\text{”}\}$. Concerning Task 3, the subject and object types of relation $r \in R_i$ are strictly required to be Gene and Disease. $R_i = \{\text{“}LOF\text{”}, \text{“}GOF\text{”}, \text{“}REG\text{”}, \text{“}COM\text{”}\}$ is a set of Gene-Disease associated relations.

4 Method

In this section, we describe our model designed for AGAC tasks. The overall structure of the model is presented in Fig. 1. The model architecture contains BERT Encoder [1], Partition Filter Encoder (PFE) [28] and Hierarchical Global Pointer Network (HGPN). BERT is used to encode contextual representation of each token in input sentence. The encoder of Partition Filter Network is applied to generate three task-specific features, ensuring sufficient task interaction and information sharing. HGPN is a two-layer stacked Global Pointer (GP) [16] that incorporates the message-passing mechanism for better relation reasoning. GP, a token-pair linking module, is the basic unit for entity and relation prediction. During training, we propose a simple but effective approach to integrate multi-hop relation paths that experimentally contribute to implicit relation inference.

4.1 BERT Encoder

The BERT model is a multi-layer bidirectional Transformer encoder [18] based on self-attention mechanism. BERT is pre-trained with two unsupervised tasks

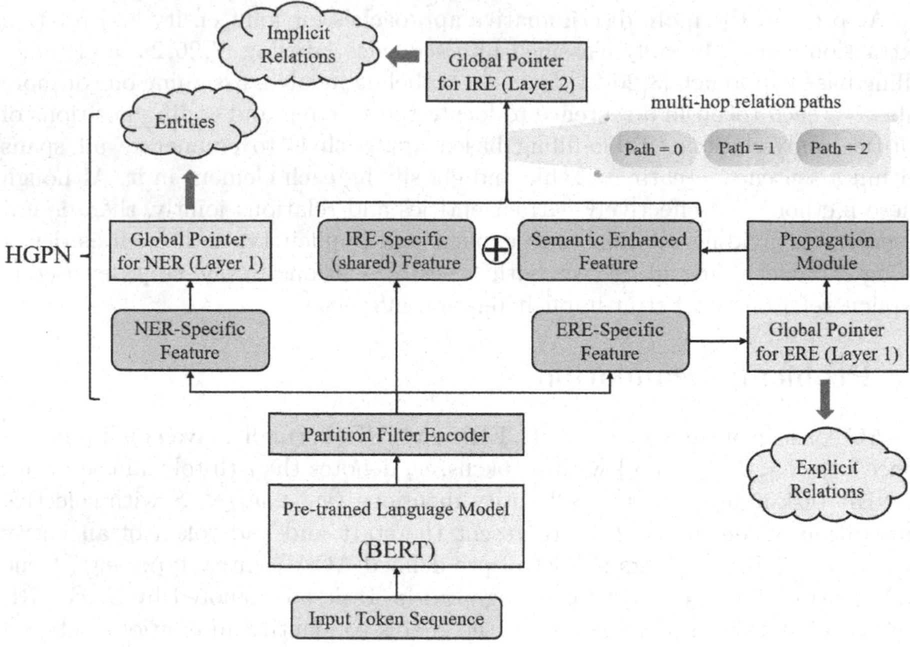

Fig. 1. The overall structure of the proposed model.

i.e., masked language model and next sentence prediction, on large-scale unannotated text datasets. The pre-trained model is then fine-turned to adapt to different downstream tasks, a process known as transfer learning. Given an input token sequence $s = w_1, w_2, \ldots, w_L$, after 12 stacked self-attention blocks, the output of BERT is a contextual representation sequence $H = h_1, h_2, \ldots, h_L$. In addition, some domain-specific language models based on BERT or its variants (such as BioBERT [8] or BioRoBERTa [9]) are pre-trained on large-scale biomedical corpora e.g., PubMed abstracts and MIMIC-III [5]. These biomedical pre-trained models contain more biomedical knowledge and can be transferred more effectively to biomedical-related tasks with minimal task-specific architecture modifications.

4.2 Partition Filter Encoder (PFE)

The encoder of Partition Filter Network is a recurrent feature encoder and is used to generate task-specific features based on shared input sequence H. At each time step, this module follows two sub-steps, partition and filter. PFE first partitions each neuron into task-specific partitions and inter-task shared partition, according to its contribution to individual tasks, and then different partitions are combined to filter task-irrelevant information.

Partition. For each time step t, similar to LSTM, a hidden state and a cell state with history information are denoted by h_t and c_t. In addition, given input token x_t, a candidate cell $\tilde{c}_t$ is calculated through linear transformation and activation function:

$$\tilde{c}_t = tanh\left(Linear\left([x_t; h_{t-1}]\right)\right) \tag{1}$$

Entity gate $\tilde{e}$ and relation gate $\tilde{r}$ are leveraged for neuron partition. The gates are calculated using cummax activation function $cummax(\cdot) = cumsum(softmax(\cdot))$ as following:

$$\begin{aligned} \tilde{e} &= cummax\left(Linear\left([x_t; h_{t-1}]\right)\right) \\ \tilde{r} &= 1 - cummax\left(Linear\left([x_t; h_{t-1}]\right)\right) \end{aligned} \tag{2}$$

Two gates naturally divide neurons for current candidate cell state $\tilde{c}_t$ and historical cell state c_{t-1}, respectively into three partitions in the same manner. The calculation for c_{t-1} is shown in Eq. (3). Three partitions include two task partitions, namely entity partition $\rho_{e,c_{t-1}}$ and relation partition $\rho_{r,c_{t-1}}$, storing intra-task information, as well as one shared partition $\rho_{s,c_{t-1}}$ to store inter-task information that is valuable to both NER and RE tasks.

$$\begin{aligned} \rho_{s,c_{t-1}} &= \tilde{e}_{c_{t-1}} \circ \tilde{r}_{c_{t-1}} \\ \rho_{e,c_{t-1}} &= \tilde{e}_{c_{t-1}} - \rho_{s,c_{t-1}} \\ \rho_{r,c_{t-1}} &= \tilde{r}_{c_{t-1}} - \rho_{s,c_{t-1}} \end{aligned} \tag{3}$$

Finally, each type of partition from both target cells are aggregated to form three partitioned results: ρ_e, ρ_r and ρ_s through Eq. (4).

$$\rho = \rho_{c_{t-1}} \circ c_{t-1} + \rho_{c_t} \circ \tilde{c}_t \tag{4}$$

Filter. Information in entity partition and shared partition are combined to form entity memory denoted by μ_e, where $\mu_e = \rho_e + \rho_s$. Information in relation partition ρ_r is assumed to be irrelevant or even harmful to NER task and thus, is filtered out. The same logic applies to relation memory $\mu_r = \rho_r + \rho_s$. The shared memory $\mu_s = \rho_s$ is evenly accessible to both entity memory and relation memory, ensuring balanced interaction between different tasks. At last, three memories are used to form cell state c_t and hidden state h_t, which will be the input to next time step.

$$\begin{aligned} c_t &= LayerNorm\left(Linear\left([\mu_{e,t}; \mu_{r,t}; \mu_{s,t}]\right)\right) \\ h_t &= tanh\left(c_t\right) \end{aligned} \tag{5}$$

In Eq. (5), layer normalization is applied to prevent gradient explosion and stabilize the training process. These three memory blocks μ_e, μ_r and μ_s are further activated and combined with corresponding global representation to form task-specific features h_e, h_r and h_s, where h_e and h_r are regarded as feature representations for NER and ERE tasks. Since shared feature h_s contains rich information related to both entity and explicit relations, h_s is considered as part of the input for IRE task.

4.3 Hierarchical Global Pointer Network (HGPN)

Analogous to the idea of TPLinker [21], we formulate joint entity and relation extraction as a type-specific table-filling problem. Token-pair linking module is used to score each element in the table, and handshaking tagging schema is referenced for decoding relational triples.

We adopt the architecture of GP as the basic unit for token-pair linking module. However, almost all such modules, including GP, score tables in parallel, which means the scores for different typed tables are generated independently, and there is no interaction between tables, except for partially shared inputs. To ease this problem, we propose HGPN, a two-layer stacked GP with interlayer propagation module, to enable explicit relational message-passing with rich text information. The intuition behind this structure is to score tables in a predefined order, so that implicit relations can be scored based on the results of first-extracted explicit relations in a supervised manner.

In HGPN, the first layer extracts entities and explicit relations, while the second layer corresponds to implicit relations. Moreover, we consider the results of explicit relations naturally form a graph-structured shallow semantic network. For each token in the graph, HGPN aims to aggregate valuable relation signals from neighbors through the message-passing paradigm to learn shallow semantic enhanced representation. This enhanced feature is further concatenated with the initial features h_s of Task 3, being fed to the second GP layer as a whole. We introduce the tagging framework, the details of basic token-pair linking unit and the interlayer propagation module in the following three paragraphs.

Token Pair Tagging Method. AGAC tasks are deconstructed into $|E| + |R_e| + |R_i|$ table-filling tasks, where $|x|$ denotes the number of elements in the set x. Each table-filling task builds a $L \times L$ scoring matrix, where L is the length of input sentence. For each AGAC entity type $k \in E$, we fill out a table whose element $e^k_{i,j}$ represents the score of a token-pair (w_i, w_j) with type k. Each token-pair (w_i, w_j) represents an entity span starting with token w_i and ending with w_j. The similar logic goes for element $r^l_{i,j}$ in relation-specific table, where w_i and w_j represent the starting token of subject and object entity with relation type $l \in R_e \cup R_i$. In this way, we can decode the relational triples $\langle w_x, w_y, l, w_m, w_n \rangle$ by querying multi-tables for token-pairs that satisfy following conditions:

$$e^{k_s}_{x,y} \geq \lambda_e; \quad e^{k_o}_{m,n} \geq \lambda_e; \quad r^l_{x,m} \geq \lambda_r \tag{6}$$

where λ_e and λ_r are the threshold for prediction, both are set to 0 by default. Particularly, in Task 3, the entity type k_s and k_o are strictly required to be Gene and Disease.

Token Pair Linking Unit. Given a task-specific feature $H = h_1, h_2, \ldots, h_L$, for each token-pair (w_i, w_j), two feedforward layers are used to map the head and tail features h_i and h_j into low-dimensional vectors $q_{i,a}$ and $k_{j,a}$ as following:

$$\begin{aligned} q_{i,a} &= W_{q,a}h_i + b_{q,a} \\ k_{j,a} &= W_{k,a}h_j + b_{k,a} \end{aligned} \tag{7}$$

where $W_{q,a}$ and $W_{k,a}$ are parameter matrixes, as well as $b_{q,a}$ and $b_{k,a}$ are bias vectors for specific type α to be learned during training. Then, the score of the token-pair that leverages the relative positions through a multiplicative attention mechanism, is calculated by Eq. (8).

$$S_\alpha(i,j) = (R_i q_{i,a})^T (R_j k_{j,a}) \tag{8}$$

Rotary position embedding [15] is applied into the score calculation, which satisfies $R_i^T R_j = R_{j-1}$.

Propagation Module. To propagate relational information among tokens, one approach is to employ a teacher forcing strategy during training, i.e., using the golden graph structure constructed by real relation labels. But this strategy inevitably causes exposure bias problem, which leads to error accumulation during inference. To avoid this, we found that the scoring matrixes in GP can be regarded as a fully-connected graph. By assigning different weights to the edges based on the internal scores, the golden graph structure can be fitted approximately.

Specifically, for each token i, the weight coefficients w_{ij}^a with one of its neighbor nodes (tokens) j is the normalization across all scores of i's neighbors (including i) using softmax function.

$$w_{ij}^a = softmax_j\left(S_\alpha(i,j)\right) = \frac{\exp\left(LeakyReLU\left(S_\alpha(i,j)\right)\right)}{\sum_{k\in 1\sim L}\exp\left(LeakyReLU\left(S_\alpha(i,k)\right)\right)} \tag{9}$$

Next, the normalized weight coefficients are used to propagate information among nodes to enhance the signal of shallow semantic relations and update token representations.

$$h_{(r',i)}^a = \sum_{k\in 1\sim L} w_{ik}^a \cdot h_{(r,k)} \tag{10}$$

Inspired by multi-head attention [18], we consider each type of explicit relation as an attention head. Features of each head are concatenated, resulting in the following shallow semantic enhanced token representation $h_{(r',i)}$ for i-th token in the input sequence, where $\|$ denotes concatenation operator.

$$h_{(r',i)} = \|_{l\in R_e} h_{(r',i)}^l \tag{11}$$

Finally, $h_{r'}$ is further concatenated with Task 3's initial features h_s, generated from PFE, to form a whole input for next GP layer.

4.4 Training Details

Since the matrix of each typed table is extremely sparse, we use Class Imbalance Loss [16] during training. The total loss is calculated as the sum of losses from all task tables:

$$\log\left(1+\sum_{(i,j)\in\Omega_{neg}^{a}} e^{-s_a^{(i,j)}}\right)+\log\left(1+\sum_{(i,j)\in\Omega_{pos}^{a}} e^{s_a(i,j)}\right) \quad (12)$$

where (i,j) represent a token-pair (w_i, w_j), Ω_{neg}^{a} represents a collection of token-pairs that do not belong to type a, Ω_{pos}^{a} represents a collection of token-pairs whose entity type or relation type is a. In particular, formula (12) is a simplified version, when the threshold λ_e and λ_r are both 0.

In addition, we explore a method to integrate multi-hop relation paths for better relation inference, without any modification of model structure. From the perspective of graph, the inputs of the second GP layer, h_s and $h_{r'}$, represent relational information under different meta-paths, whose lengths are 0 and 1 respectively. To leverage higher-order meta-path, e.g., for $\forall A \in R_e$, $\forall B \in R_e$ ($A = B$ is allowed), we generate new labels for those entity pairs that conform to the 2-order meta-path "A-B" from the training dataset. All new labels are merged into the original set R_e.

Table 1. Statistics for entity types in the AGAC training set.

Entity Name	Count	Percentage
Disease	415	17.12%
Gene	475	19.60%
Protein	60	2.48%
Enzyme	19	0.78%
Variation	569	23.47%
MPA	200	8.25%
Interaction	7	0.29%
Pathway	14	0.58%
CPA	56	2.31%
Reg	398	16.42%
PosReg	83	3.42%
NegReg	128	5.28%
Overall	2424	100%

5 Experiment

In this section, we provide data distribution details of AGAC dataset, the leaderboard performance and an analysis of the effect of proposed model.

5.1 AGAC Dataset

The AGAC dataset consists of 2,250 PubMed abstracts, with 250 used for model training and 2,000 for testing and final evaluation. The statistical analysis of the AGAC dataset reveals the challenges of few-shot samples and class imbalance. Table 1 illustrates the distribution of 12 entity types in the training set, some of which have less than 20 examples e.g., interaction, pathway and enzyme (less than 1%). In addition to the previously mentioned LOF and GOF, the implicit relation types also include Regulation (REG) and Complex (COM). REG indicates the function change that is either neutral or unknown, while COM with only 6 examples, refers to those complex function changes that cannot be described by other relation types. The distribution of relation types is presented in Table 2, from which we can find the amount ratio of REG and COM reaches an imbalance of 227:6. The aforementioned challenges are not the research objects in this work, although they are non-ignorable and will affect the performance of the algorithms.

Table 2. Statistics for explicit and implicit relation types in the AGAC training set.

Relation Name - Explicit	Count	Percentage
ThemeOf	1288	66.12%
CauseOf	660	33.88%
Overall	1948	100%
Relation Name - Implicit	Count	Percentage
LOF	63	19.75%
GOF	23	7.21%
REG	227	71.16%
COM	6	1.88%
Overall	319	100%

5.2 Experimental Setup

We randomly split the 250 labeled abstracts into train and development datasets with the ratio of 4:1. The training set is utilized to learn model parameters, while the development set is utilized to select optimal hyperparameters. We generated position information for the entities in the explicit relation triples using a heuristic algorithm, as this information is not provided in the original dataset for Task 3. The AGAC track is evaluated by the micro-F1 score of Task 1 and Task 2, as well as the macro-F1 score of Task 3. We employed a five-fold cross-validation approach to apply ensemble learning to multiple models and evaluate the final performance of our proposed method on the test set.

5.3 Implementation and Hyperparameters

We conducted experiments using various versions of the BERT model, including two base-level PubMedBERT [2] (one pretrained from scratch using PubMed abstracts, and the other pretrained on a combination of PubMedCentral (PMC) full-text articles and PubMed abstracts), and two base-level and one large-level BioRoBERTa models [9] pretrained on PubMed, PMC and MIMIC-III with different training strategies.

For all of these pre-trained models, we employed the same set of following hyperparameters without any further fine-tuning. Each training sample is pruned to at most 512 tokens. We used a batch size of 16 and employed the hierarchical learning rate in the training process with Adam optimizer [6], using a learning rate of $1e-5$ for pre-trained weights and $1e-4$ for other weights. We trained for at most 60 epochs with early stopping strategy based on the performance of development set. Training stops when the F1 score on the development set fails to improve for 10 consecutive epochs or the maximum number of epochs has been reached. The hidden vector dimensions are set to 384 (512 for the large model) and 128 for PFE and HGPN respectively.

To ensure the best performance, we selected different epochs that can achieve the highest F1-score on corresponding tasks. For the first two tasks, we conducted ensemble learning through hard-voting by selecting three models with the highest F1 scores from five different pre-trained models for each fold during the five-fold cross-validation (totally, $3 \times 5 = 15$ models per task for ensemble). For Task 3, we first took the union set of multiple results predicted within five-fold cross-validation for each pre-trained model, as a single model tends to have high precision but low recall. Then we performed a hard voting on the prediction results of multiple pre-trained models.

5.4 Results

Table 3. Model results in development set with different pre-trained models.

Model	Task 1	Task 2	Task 3				
	F1	F1	LOF_{F1}	GOF_{F1}	REG_{F1}	COM_{F1}	Macro-F1
$PubMed_{abstract}$	61.60	48.97	**47.16**	35.78	8.00	0.00	22.73
$PubMed_{fulltext}$	60.22	48.41	40.50	**37.56**	0.00	0.00	19.52
$BioRo_{distill-align}$	62.44	**50.23**	44.57	35.36	**13.71**	0.00	**23.41**
$BioRo_{train-longer}$	61.59	49.47	45.81	34.14	13.08	0.00	23.26
$BioRo_{large-Voc}$	**62.66**	49.01	43.98	33.44	13.00	0.00	22.60

Table 3 presents the results of various pre-trained models according to the average scores obtained through five-fold cross-validation in the development set. The large-level BioRoBERTa model yields the highest performance in Task 1, with an F1 score of 62.66%. The base-level BioRoBERTa that distilled from the large one with additional alignment objective, achieves the best F1 score of 50.23% for Task 2. In addition, the F1 scores for each relation type are presented in detail in Task 3. The experimental results show our model struggles with few-shot learning, as it fails to learn COM from only 6 samples. Meanwhile, although

REG has a larger number of samples, its F1 score is much lower than that of LOF and GOF. It is probably due to the semantic definition of REG itself (a neutral function change between GOF and LOF), which makes it more difficult to learn. The highest F1 score in Task 3 is 23.41%.

Table 4. F1 score for each type in test set of AGAC Task 1&2.

Entity Name	F1	Entity Name	F1	Relation Name	F1
Disease	0.50	Pathway	0.25	CauseOf	0.36
Gene	0.63	CPA	0.09	ThemeOf	0.28
Protein	0.26	Reg	0.55	Overall	**0.31**
Enzyme	0.18	PosReg	0.63		
Variation	0.52	NegReg	0.62		
MPA	0.39	Overall	**0.52**		
Interaction	0.13				

Table 4 summarizes the final evaluation results for Task 1 and Task 2. Our model performs poorly on recognizing three entity types i.e., interaction, pathway and enzyme. It may be due to the lack of training instances for those entities. The overall micro-F1 scores in Task 1 and Task 2 reach 52% and 31% respectively. As shown in Table 5, the macro-F1 score of IRE task on the test set increases by 6.84% compared to that on the development set, reaching 30.25%. One of the reasons is we combined the results of multiple models by taking the union set of their predictions.

Table 5. Precision (P), Recall (R) and F1 scores in test set of AGAC Task 3.

Relation Name	P	R	F1
LOF	0.77	0.36	0.50
GOF	1.00	0.14	0.25
REG	0.52	0.41	0.46
COM	0.00	0.00	0.00
Overall (Macro)	0.57	0.23	**0.30**

5.5 Ablation Study

To evaluate the validity of each component of our approach, we conducted ablation experiments on the development set using base-level PubMedBERT pretrained from PubMed abstracts. As illustrated in Table 6, incorporating PFE can effectively enhance model's performance, suggesting that information sharing among different tasks can not only alleviate the selective annotation problem, but also enable each task to benefit from each other. Additionally, the structure of HGPN is effective for implicit relation inference, and it increases the F1 score by 2.11%. Experiments further demonstrate that integrating the labels of 2-order relation paths contributes to relation inference.

Table 6. Ablation study in development set.

Model	Task 1	Task 2	Task 3
PubMed$_{\text{abstract}}$	61.60	48.97	22.73
w/o PFE	59.85	47.13	21.17
w/o HGPN	/	/	20.62
w/o 2-order meta-path	/	/	22.29

6 Conclusion and Discussion

In this paper, we proposed a unified end-to-end model that can simultaneously achieve three AGAC tasks. A novel HGPN with propagation module is designed for implicit relation inference based on explicit relations. Additionally, our experiments demonstrate that PFE can effectively generate task-specific features and model the interactions between entities and relations, alleviating the problem of selective annotation. However, our model does not perform well on target type with few-shot samples. In future research, it would be valuable to explore strategies for data augmentation or integrate few-shot learning techniques.

References

1. Devlin, J., Chang, M.W., Lee, K., Toutanova, K.: BERT: pre-training of deep bidirectional transformers for language understanding. In: Proceedings of the 2019 Conference of the North American Chapter of the Association for Computational Linguistics: Human Language Technologies, Volume 1 (Long and Short Papers), Minneapolis, Minnesota, pp. 4171–4186. Association for Computational Linguistics (2019)
2. Gu, Y., et al.: Domain-specific language model pretraining for biomedical natural language processing. ACM Trans. Comput. Healthcare **3**(1), 2:1–2:23 (2021)
3. Gupta, P., Schütze, H., Andrassy, B.: Table filling multi-task recurrent neural network for joint entity and relation extraction. In: Proceedings of COLING 2016, the 26th International Conference on Computational Linguistics: Technical Papers, Osaka, Japan, pp. 2537–2547. The COLING 2016 Organizing Committee (2016)
4. Hunter, L., Cohen, K.B.: Biomedical language processing: what's beyond PubMed? Mol. Cell **21**(5), 589–594 (2006)
5. Johnson, A.E.W., et al.: MIMIC-III, a freely accessible critical care database. Sci. Data **3**(1), 160035 (2016)
6. Kingma, D.P., Ba, J.: Adam: a method for stochastic optimization. In: Bengio, Y., LeCun, Y. (eds.) 3rd International Conference on Learning Representations, ICLR 2015, San Diego, CA, USA, 7–9 May 2015, Conference Track Proceedings (2015)

7. Lample, G., Ballesteros, M., Subramanian, S., Kawakami, K., Dyer, C.: Neural architectures for named entity recognition. In: Proceedings of the 2016 Conference of the North American Chapter of the Association for Computational Linguistics: Human Language Technologies, San Diego, California, pp. 260–270. Association for Computational Linguistics (2016)
8. Lee, J., et al.: BioBERT: a pre-trained biomedical language representation model for biomedical text mining. Bioinformatics **36**(4), 1234–1240 (2020)
9. Lewis, P., Ott, M., Du, J., Stoyanov, V.: Pretrained language models for biomedical and clinical tasks: understanding and extending the state-of-the-art. In: Proceedings of the 3rd Clinical Natural Language Processing Workshop, pp. 146–157. Association for Computational Linguistics, Online (2020)
10. Li, D., Xiong, Y., Hu, B., Tang, B., Peng, W., Chen, Q.: Drug knowledge discovery via multi-task learning and pre-trained models. BMC Med. Inform. Decis. Mak. **21**(9), 251 (2021)
11. Li, Y.H., et al.: Therapeutic target database update 2018: enriched resource for facilitating bench-to-clinic research of targeted therapeutics. Nucleic Acids Res. **46**(D1), D1121–D1127 (2018)
12. Liu, F., Zheng, X., Wang, B., Kiefe, C.: DeepGeneMD: a joint deep learning model for extracting gene mutation-disease knowledge from PubMed literature. In: Proceedings of the 5th Workshop on BioNLP Open Shared Tasks, Hong Kong, China, pp. 77–83. Association for Computational Linguistics (2019)
13. Ouyang, S., Yao, X., Wang, Y., Peng, Q., He, Z., Xia, J.: An overview of the text mining task for "gene-disease" association semantics. J. Med. Inform. **43**(12), 6–9 (2022)
14. Ouyang, S., Yao, X., Wang, Y., Peng, Q., He, Z., Xia, J.: Text mining task for "gene-disease" association semantics in CHIP 2022. In: Health Information Processing: 8th China Conference. CHIP 2022, pp. 21–23. Springer, Cham (2022)
15. Su, J., Lu, Y., Pan, S., Wen, B., Liu, Y.: Roformer: Enhanced transformer with rotary position embedding. arXiv preprint arXiv:2104.09864 (2021)
16. Su, J., et al.: Global Pointer: Novel Efficient Span-based Approach for Named Entity Recognition. arXiv preprint arXiv:2208.03054 (2022)
17. Thillaisundaram, A., Togia, T.: Biomedical relation extraction with pre-trained language representations and minimal task-specific architecture. In: Proceedings of the 5th Workshop on BioNLP Open Shared Tasks, Hong Kong, China, pp. 84–89. Association for Computational Linguistics (2019)
18. Vaswani, A., et al.: Attention is all you need. In: Advances in Neural Information Processing Systems, vol. 30. Curran Associates, Inc. (2017)
19. Veličković, P., Cucurull, G., Casanova, A., Romero, A., Liò, P., Bengio, Y.: Graph attention networks. In: International Conference on Learning Representations (2018)
20. Wadden, D., Wennberg, U., Luan, Y., Hajishirzi, H.: Entity, relation, and event extraction with contextualized span representations. In: Proceedings of the 2019 Conference on Empirical Methods in Natural Language Processing and the 9th International Joint Conference on Natural Language Processing (EMNLP-IJCNLP), Hong Kong, China, pp. 5784–5789. Association for Computational Linguistics (2019)
21. Wang, Y., Yu, B., Zhang, Y., Liu, T., Zhu, H., Sun, L.: TPLinker: single-stage joint extraction of entities and relations through token pair linking. In: Proceedings of the 28th International Conference on Computational Linguistics, Barcelona, Spain, pp. 1572–1582. International Committee on Computational Linguistics (Online) (2020)

22. Wang, Y., et al.: Guideline design of an active gene annotation corpus for the purpose of drug repurposing. In: 2018 11th International Congress on Image and Signal Processing, BioMedical Engineering and Informatics (CISP-BMEI), pp. 1–5 (2018)
23. Wang, Y., Zhou, K., Gachloo, M., Xia, J.: An overview of the active gene annotation corpus and the BioNLP OST 2019 AGAC track tasks. In: Proceedings of the 5th Workshop on BioNLP Open Shared Tasks, Hong Kong, China, pp. 62–71. Association for Computational Linguistics (2019)
24. Wang, Y., et al.: An active gene annotation corpus and its application on anti-epilepsy drug discovery. In: 2019 IEEE International Conference on Bioinformatics and Biomedicine (BIBM), pp. 512–519 (2019)
25. Wang, Z.Y., Zhang, H.Y.: Rational drug repositioning by medical genetics. Nat. Biotechnol. **31**(12), 1080–1082 (2013)
26. Wei, Z., Su, J., Wang, Y., Tian, Y., Chang, Y.: A novel cascade binary tagging framework for relational triple extraction. In: Proceedings of the 58th Annual Meeting of the Association for Computational Linguistics, pp. 1476–1488. Association for Computational Linguistics, Online (2020)
27. Wishart, D.S., et al.: DrugBank 5.0: a major update to the DrugBank database for 2018. Nucleic Acids Res. **46**(D1), D1074–D1082 (2018)
28. Yan, Z., Zhang, C., Fu, J., Zhang, Q., Wei, Z.: A partition filter network for joint entity and relation extraction. In: Proceedings of the 2021 Conference on Empirical Methods in Natural Language Processing, Punta Cana, Dominican Republic, pp. 185–197. Association for Computational Linguistics, Online (2021)
29. Zheng, S., Wang, F., Bao, H., Hao, Y., Zhou, P., Xu, B.: Joint extraction of entities and relations based on a novel tagging scheme. In: Proceedings of the 55th Annual Meeting of the Association for Computational Linguistics (Volume 1: Long Papers), Vancouver, Canada, pp. 1227–1236. Association for Computational Linguistics (2017)
30. Zhou, K., et al.: Bridging heterogeneous mutation data to enhance disease gene discovery. Brief. Bioinform. **22**(5), bbab079 (2021)
31. Zong, H., et al.: Overview of technology evaluation dataset for medical multimodal information extraction. J. Med. Inform. **43**(12), 2–5 (2022)

A Knowledge-Based Data Augmentation Framework for Few-Shot Biomedical Information Extraction

Xin Su, Chuang Cheng, Kuo Yang(✉), and Xuezhong Zhou(✉)

School of Computer and Information Technology, Beijing Jiaotong University, Beijing 100044, China
{21140085,21125146,yangkuo,xzzhou}@bjtu.edu.cn

Abstract. There are a lot of biomedical knowledge hidden in the massive scientific clinical literature. These knowledge exist in an unstructured form and is difficult to extract automatically. Natural language processing makes it possible to mine these knowledge automatically. At present, most information extraction models need enough data to achieve good performance. Due to the scarcity of high-quality biomedical labeled data, it is still difficult to extract biomedical literature accurately in the case of few samples. This paper describes our participation in the task 1 of the "China Health Information Processing Conference" (CHIP 2022). We proposes a knowledge-based data augmentation framework to achieve data expansion to overcome the scarcity of training data. The experimental results show that after data augmentation, the $F1$ *score* of named entity recognition using BioBERT-BiLSTM-CRF reaches 0.58 and the $F1$ *score* of relation extraction using TDEER reaches 0.6. Finally, we win the second place, which validates the performance of our approach.

Keywords: Few-Shot · Data Augmentation · Named Entity Recognition · Relation Extraction

1 Introduction

With the rapid development of biomedical research, the scientific literature has grown exponentially [36]. The literature contains rich medical information, which can provide professional data and knowledge for scientific research. However, this information hidden in them exist in an unstructured form, which cannot be used effectively and hinder the discovery of medical knowledge. Therefore, it is necessary to use information extraction technology [24] to automatically mine and extract valuable information from massive literature.

The core technologies of information extraction include named entity recognition (NER) and relation extraction (RE). NER is mainly used to extract entity information in text, such as disease, gene, symptom, etc. RE can further extract

X. Su and C. Cheng—Contributed equally to this work.

B. Tang et al. (Eds.): CHIP 2022, CCIS 1773, pp. 29–40, 2023.
https://doi.org/10.1007/978-981-99-4826-0_3

the biomedical semantic relation between entities [30]. Currently, NER and RE tasks mainly use deep learning methods. These methods do not require manual construction of features and show high accuracy [26], but usually require a large amount of labeled data for training. However, in the biomedical domain, labeled data requires professional knowledge and usually requires experts to annotate and review. So it will take much time and effort [25], leading to data low-resources.

The 8th China Health Information Processing Conference (CHIP 2022), focusing on "Real World Research and Digital Therapy", organizes five tasks. Among them, task 1 is a text mining task for "Gene-Disease" association semantics, which includes trigger word entity recognition and "Gene, Regulation type, Disease" triplet extraction. The task of trigger word entity recognition is NER in the traditional sense, which is used to identify 12 types of molecular objects related to "Gene-Disease" and their trigger word entities, including Variation (Var), Molecular Physiological Activity (MPA), Interaction, Pathway, Cell Physiological Activity (CPA), Regulation (Reg), Positive Regulation (PosReg), Negative Regulation (NegReg), Disease, Gene, Protein and Enzyme. The triple extraction of "Gene, Regulation type and Disease" is a RE task, which extracts the regulatory types of "Gene-Disease" association mechanisms. The regulatory type includes four semantic descriptions of mutant genes: loss of function (LOF), gain of function (GOF), regulation of function (REG), and complex change of function (COM) [27,28].

This paper conducts research on trigger word entity recognition and "Gene, Regulatory type, Disease" triplet extraction method on the few-shot dataset provided by the sponsor. To solve the problem of low resources, this paper proposes a data augmentation framework based on external knowledge, which can easily expand training samples and overcome the scarcity of labeled data. For the trigger word entity recognition task, this paper uses a BioBERT-BiLSTM-CRF model, which can accurately extract trigger word entities and achieves 0.5654 of $F1$ *score* on the test set. After using data augmentation, the $F1$ *score* reaches 0.5789. For the triplet extraction task of "Gene, Regulatory type, Disease", this paper adopts TDEER, a state-of-the-art relation extraction model, achieves 0.6 of $F1$ *score* with the augmented dataset.

2 Related Work

2.1 Named Entity Recognition

Biomedical named entity recognition (BioNER) methods are roughly divided into three classes: rule-based methods [13,33], machine learning methods and deep learning methods. Specifically, rule-based methods use term-matching strategies to find entities in the text that also appear in the lexicon, so the method is difficult to generalize to identify entities outside the vocabulary. Machine learning methods treat NER as a classification problem and train statistical models such as decision tree or support vector machine (SVM) [8,15], or

Markov model-based sequence labeling models such as HMM and CRF [4,17,20] to achieve the goal. In recent years, deep learning methods have been applied to NER. For example, Lee et al. [21] released BioBERT to train the BERT model on biomedical article texts from PubMed, improving the performance of BioNER tasks. Beltagy et al. [1] proposed a BERT-based pre-trained contextualized embedding model for scientific text, named SciBERT. SciBERT achieves better performance on BC5CDR [22] and NCBI-Disease [9] datasets.

2.2 Relation Extraction

Biomedical relation extraction (BioRE) is mainly oriented to medical literature, such as disease-gene, drug-target and other relation types. It mainly includes three classes: rule-based methods, machine learning methods and deep learning methods. In the rule-based methods, rules are typically defined manually by domain experts. For example, Hakenberg et al. [12] defined and extracted syntactic patterns learned from tagged examples and match them to texts to detect protein-protein interactions. Classification techniques based on machine learning are also widely used RE methods in the biomedical domain. For example, Rink et al. [32] applied SVM to extract the relation between medical records and treatments. Furthermore, Bundschus et al. [3] proposed a CRF based classification method. It was a supervised machine learning approach, which used syntactic and semantic features of context to identify the relations between gene and disease. In recent years, deep learning-based relation extraction methods have gradually developed. Hsieh et al. [14] proposed an RNN-based method to capture long-term relations between words to identify protein interaction relations. Tuan et al. [19] proposed a GCN model combined with an external knowledge base to perform relation extraction on the two corpora of BioRelEx [16] and ADE [11].

2.3 Data Augmentation

Currently, most deep learning-based models require a large amount of annotated corpus to achieve good performance. However, high-quality labeled data is scarce in biomedical domain. Thus how to train a better-performance information extraction model with few annotated data is significant. To alleviate the scarcity of biomedical labeled data, researchers have introduced some strategies, such as distant supervision, data augmentation and so on. Su et al. [37] proposed a distant supervision model to augment data for relation extraction. This method assumes that the same entity pair has the same relation in all sentences to augment data for each relation from an external corpus, but this method may generate some data noise [29,41]. Data augmentation can easily expand training data, including strategies such as word replacement, random insertion, exchange or deletion, reverse translation. Wei et al. [39] proposed an Easy Data Augmentation (EDA) method to improve the performance of sentence classification. Dai et al. [5] applied traditional data augmentation methods to NER and made a comprehensive analysis and comparison. Ding et al. [7] designed a language generation model for data augmentation, applied to both supervised and semi supervised scenarios. In biomedical NLP task, Skreta et al. [35] used word-embedding data augmentation to embed the Unified Medical Language System (UMLS) concept for the medical abbreviation disambiguation task.

3 Our Models and Methods

An overview of our method is shown in Fig. 1, which mainly includes two parts: the first one is data augmentation, and the other is the downstream tasks of NER and RE. In the data augmentation part, the article abstracts are firstly split into sentences, which are used as input. Then, we query diseases and gene entities from external biomedical knowledge bases (KBs) such as MalaCards [31], UMLS [2], and GeneCards [34] to extract their synonyms. Finally, we replace entities in the original sentence with synonyms and get the augmented training corpus. In the information extraction part, the downstream tasks of NER and RE are done on the training set after data augmentation.

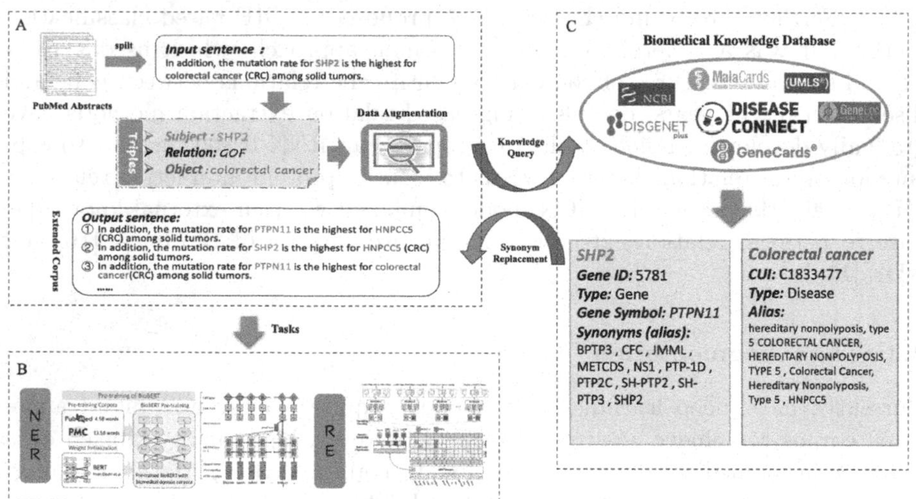

Fig. 1. The overview of our method. (A) Data preprocessing and augmentation. (B) Specific process of data augmentation method based on external KBs. (C) Downstream tasks. NER and RE tasks are done on the augmented dataset.

3.1 Data Augmentation Method

For the few-shot problem in this study, we improve the original EDA [39] method to achieve data expansion of training samples and overcome the scarcity of labeled data. In order to apply EDA to the biomedical domain, this paper identify entity concepts from the external KBs and replace them with synonyms in the sentences. That is, for disease and gene entities, we extract their semantic types and synonym information from external KBs such as MalaCards and GeneCards etc. As is shown in Fig. 1, the process is divided into three steps: 1) Randomly select candidate sentences in the training data, query entity synonyms from KBs; 2) Randomly select entity aliases according to a certain probability P ($P = 0.5$); 3) Randomly perform synonym replacement in the selected sentences to generate a new sentence, which is added to the original dataset.

3.2 Named Entity Recognition Models

For the trigger word entity recognition task, this paper uses the BioBERT-BiLSTM-CRF model. The model is mainly divided into three modules. 1) Use the pre-trained language model BioBERT to obtain the word vector representation of the input text; 2) Input word vectors into the BiLSTM module to learn sequence features; 3) Use the CRF model to decode the label.

BioBERT. It is a pre-trained language representation model for biomedical domain, which was proposed by Lee et al. [21] in 2020. It is based on the model structure of BERT [6], initialized with the same weights as BERT, and trained on biomedical domain corpus (PubMed abstracts and PMC full texts). BioBERT performs better than BERT in various biomedical information extraction tasks.

BiLSTM. Graves et al. [10] proposed BiLSTM (Bidirectional Long-Short Term Memory). The model consists of forward LSTM and backward LSTM. Compared with LSTM, BiLSTM can better learn bidirectional semantic information. For the hidden layer output h_t at time t, BiLSTM obtains the final output by splicing the features in two directions, namely:

$$h_t = \begin{bmatrix} \overrightarrow{h_t} \\ \overleftarrow{h_t} \end{bmatrix} \tag{1}$$

CRF. It was proposed by Lafferty et al. [18] in 2001 and was a discriminant probability model. CRF can be abstracted as a probability distribution model $P(Y|X)$, which represents a Markov random field of another set of output random variables Y under the condition of a given set of input random variables X. In information extraction tasks, CRF is often used as a decoder for NER. It can learn the dependencies between labels from the training data automatically and solve the illegal problem of label prediction by adding some rules, so as to improve the accuracy of prediction.

3.3 Relation Extraction Models

For the triplet extraction task, this paper selects some advanced relation extraction methods to compare, such as CasRel [40], TPLinker [38], PRGC [42] and TDEER [23]. Due to the need to extract triplets of "Gene-Disease", we uniformly employ BioBERT [21] as an encoder to train the datasets to evaluate their performance under the original setting. The models are as follows.

CasRel. Wei et al. [40] proposed a cascading relation extraction framework. The framework extracts the subject and regards each relation as a mapping function to match the corresponding object. Specifically, it first identifies all possible topics in a sentence. Then for each topic, apply a span-based tokenizer to identify the corresponding object according to each relation.

TPLinker. The model [38] adopts the idea of long sequence labeling and employs a token-pair linking scheme in order to extract entities and align subjects with objects under each relation. First, the whole sentence is encoded by BERT. Then the concatenated tokens are fed into a fully connected layer and the output is activated as a vector representation of the token pair. Finally, the token pairs are classified.

PRGC. It decomposes RE into three tasks: relation judgment, entity extraction, and subject-object alignment [42]. Firstly, the relation contained in the text is obtained through the relation judgment module and the impossible relation is filtered out. Then, the relation information is added to the entity extraction module, and the corresponding subject and object entities are extracted for each relation. Finally, the subject-object entities are aligned using the global entity correlation matrix obtained by the subject-object alignment module to extract the triples.

TDEER. The model [23] is divided into three steps: 1) Use the span-based entity label model to extract all subject entities and object entities; 2) Employ multi-label classification strategy to detect all correlations; 3) Iterate the subject entity and relation pairs through the translation mechanism-based decoding scheme to identify the respective object entities.

4 Experiments

4.1 Dataset

The dataset [27,28,43] is derived from CHIP 2022 task 1. Among them, the training data is 250 PubMed literature abstracts, which labels 12 types of entities including Var, MPA, Interaction, Pathway, CPA, Reg, PosReg, NegReg, Disease, Gene, Protein, Enzyme and 4 relation types including LOF, GOF, REG, and COM.

Table 1. The number of relation types before and after data augmentation in RE task.

Relation type	Train	Train (DA)	Test
COM	5	15	1
LOF	22	370	22
GOF	41	689	2
REG	150	2520	83
total	218	3594	108

Table 2. The number of entity types before and after data augmentation in NER task.

Entity type	Train	Train (DA)	Test
Var	456	747	114
Gene	386	611	87
Disease	332	646	83
Reg	321	430	78
MPA	169	223	32
NegReg	111	130	17
PosReg	69	82	15
Protein	51	63	9
CPA	44	61	12
Enzyme	18	20	1
Pathway	12	17	2
Interaction	7	12	0
total	1976	3042	450

First, this paper uses ScispaCy to split the literature abstracts, and divides them into train set and test set with a ratio of 7:3. Since the original dataset has few samples, this paper uses data augmentation method to expand the data. The statistical information of the data set before and after augmentation is shown in Table 1 and Table 2, where DA indicates that data augmentation is used.

4.2 Evaluation Indicators

The evaluation indicators of this task include *Precision* (P), *Recall* (R) and $F1$ *score* ($F1$), and the final ranking is based on $Micro - F1$. Suppose there are n types of entities (relations): $C_1, C_2, C_3, \cdots, C_n$. For entity (relation) type i, the calculation formulas of its P_i, R_i, $F1_i$ are as follows.

$$P_i = \frac{TP_i}{TP_i + FP_i} \tag{2}$$

$$R_i = \frac{TP_i}{TP_i + FN_i} \tag{3}$$

$$F1_i = \frac{2 * P_i * R_i}{P_i + R_i} \tag{4}$$

The $Micro - P$, $Micro - R$ and $Micro - F1$ of the entire task are calculated as follows.

$$Micro - P = \frac{\sum TP_i}{\sum (TP_i + FP_i)} \tag{5}$$

$$Micro - R = \frac{\sum TP_i}{\sum (TP_i + FN_i)} \tag{6}$$

$$Micro - F1 = \frac{2 * P * R}{P + R} \tag{7}$$

Among them, TP refers to the number of entity (relation) types identified by the model that are the same as the actual type, FP refers to the number of entity (relation) types recognized by the model that are different from the actual type, and FN refers to the number of entity (relation) types that are not identified in the actual type. The *Precision* measures the accuracy of the model, the *Recall* measures the completeness of the model, and the $F1$ *score* combines their results, which can more objectively evaluate the quality of the model.

4.3 Parameter Settings

In subtask 1 trigger word entity recognition, we used BioBERT-BiLSTM-CRF (BioLC) model, where the learning rate is set to 1e-5, the batch size is 16, the number of training epochs is 50 and the deep learning framework (DLF) we used is PyTorch. In the triplet extraction of subtask 3 "Gene, Regulatory type, Disease", the model we used is TDEER, where the learning rate is set to 2e-5, the batch size is 16, the number of training epochs is 100 and the DLF we used is TensorFlow. The parameters of other models compared in this paper are shown in Table 3.

Table 3. Parameters used in our experiments.

Task	Model	Learning rate	Batch size	Epoch	DLF
NER	CRF	-	16	-	PyTorch
	BiLSTM	1e-3	16	50	PyTorch
	BioLC	1e-5	16	50	PyTorch
RE	CasRel	1e-5	6	100	TensorFlow
	TPLinker	5e-5	6	100	PyTorch
	PRGC	1e-3	6	100	PyTorch
	TDEER	2e-5	6	100	TensorFlow

4.4 Results

In NER task, this paper uses three models of CRF, BiLSTM and BioLC for experimental comparison. In the RE task, this paper uses four models such as TPLinker and TDEER for experimental comparison. The experimental results are shown in Table 4.

Table 4. The results of different models on the test dataset.

Task	Model	P	R	F1
NER	CRF	0.5726	0.1578	0.2474
	BiLSTM	0.3666	0.3022	0.3313
	BioLC	0.5418	0.5911	0.5654
	BioLC (DA)	0.5714	0.5867	0.5789
RE	CasRel	0.4118	0.1308	0.1986
	TPLinker	0	0	0
	PRGC	0.3060	0.2910	0.2990
	TDEER	0.6571	0.4423	0.5287
	TDEER (DA)	0.6117	0.5888	0.6000

To verify the effectiveness of data augmentation, this paper compares the performance of different models before and after data augmentation. The experimental results are shown in Table 5. For NER task, the BioLC model performed best ($P = 0.5714$, $R = 0.5867$, $F1 = 0.5789$). After data augmentation, each model has different degrees of improvement, among which the CRF model has the most improvement (4.73%). With the increase of model complexity, the improvement rate shows a downward trend. For RE task, TDEER model achieves the highest performance with an $F1$ *score* of 0.60. After using data augmentation, the performance of each model is significantly improved, and PRGC model has the largest improvement with an rate of 70.57%.

In summary, when the dataset has fewer samples, data augmentation can be used to easily expand the data to improve the performance of information extraction model. In addition, the results also show that data augmentation can improve on different models, but when the original model has good performance, the improvement effect is not significant.

5 Discussion

In this paper, we proposed a knowledge-based data augmentation framework which extended the original EDA method for NER and RE tasks. This framework integrated UMLS, MalaCards and other KBs' knowledge into the data augmentation, expanded and generated a large amount of biomedical labeled

Table 5. Performance of data augmentation on different models.

Task	Model	F1	F1 (DA)	Improve
NER	CRF	0.2474	0.2591	4.73%
	BiLSTM	0.3313	0.3424	3.35%
	BioLC	0.5654	0.5789	2.39%
RE	CasRel	0.1986	0.3108	56.50%
	TPLinker	0	0.3048	-
	PRGC	0.299	0.51	70.57%
	TDEER	0.5287	0.6	13.49%

data. The experiment verified the feasibility and effectiveness of the data augmentation method based on external biomedical knowledge for few-shot biomedical information model. We hope to provide a certain reference for low-resource information extraction. However, the augmented dataset obtained in this paper will also enlarge the noise of the original dataset in a way. In the future, we will hope to explore the effects of different multiples of extended dataset on model performance and design individual data augmentation method according to the feature of the dataset to achieve better results.

References

1. Beltagy, I., Cohan, A., Lo, K.: Scibert: pretrained contextualized embeddings for scientific text. arXiv preprint arXiv:1903.10676 (2019)
2. Bodenreider, O.: The unified medical language system (UMLS): integrating biomedical terminology. Nucleic Acids Res. **32**(suppl_1), D267–D270 (2004)
3. Bundschus, M., Dejori, M., Stetter, M., Tresp, V., Kriegel, H.P.: Extraction of semantic biomedical relations from text using conditional random fields. BMC Bioinform. **9**(1), 1–14 (2008)
4. Chowdhury, M.F.M., Lavelli, A.: Disease mention recognition with specific features. In: Proceedings of the 2010 Workshop on Biomedical Natural Language Processing, pp. 83–90 (2010)
5. Dai, X., Adel, H.: An analysis of simple data augmentation for named entity recognition. arXiv preprint arXiv:2010.11683 (2020)
6. Devlin, J., Chang, M.W., Lee, K., Toutanova, K.: Bert: pre-training of deep bidirectional transformers for language understanding. arXiv preprint arXiv:1810.04805 (2018)
7. Ding, B., et al.: DAGA: data augmentation with a generation approach for low-resource tagging tasks. arXiv preprint arXiv:2011.01549 (2020)
8. Doan, S., Xu, H.: Recognizing medication related entities in hospital discharge summaries using support vector machine. In: Proceedings of COLING. International Conference on Computational Linguistics, vol. 2010, p. 259. NIH Public Access (2010)
9. Doğan, R.I., Leaman, R., Lu, Z.: NCBI disease corpus: a resource for disease name recognition and concept normalization. J. Biomed. Inform. **47**, 1–10 (2014)

10. Graves, A., Schmidhuber, J.: Framewise phoneme classification with bidirectional LSTM and other neural network architectures. Neural Netw. **18**(5–6), 602–610 (2005)
11. Gurulingappa, H., Rajput, A.M., Roberts, A., Fluck, J., Hofmann-Apitius, M., Toldo, L.: Development of a benchmark corpus to support the automatic extraction of drug-related adverse effects from medical case reports. J. Biomed. Inform. **45**(5), 885–892 (2012)
12. Hakenberg, J., Plake, C., Leser, U., Kirsch, H., Rebholz-Schuhmann, D.: LLL'05 challenge: genic interaction extraction-identification of language patterns based on alignment and finite state automata. In: Proceedings of the 4th Learning Language in Logic Workshop (LLL 2005), pp. 38–45 (2005)
13. Hettne, K.M., et al.: A dictionary to identify small molecules and drugs in free text. Bioinformatics **25**(22), 2983–2991 (2009)
14. Hsieh, Y.L., Chang, Y.C., Chang, N.W., Hsu, W.L.: Identifying protein-protein interactions in biomedical literature using recurrent neural networks with long short-term memory. In: Proceedings of the Eighth International Joint Conference on Natural Language Processing (Volume 2: Short Papers), pp. 240–245 (2017)
15. Isozaki, H., Kazawa, H.: Efficient support vector classifiers for named entity recognition. In: COLING 2002: The 19th International Conference on Computational Linguistics (2002)
16. Khachatrian, H., et al.: Biorelex 1.0: biological relation extraction benchmark. In: Proceedings of the 18th BioNLP Workshop and Shared Task, pp. 176–190 (2019)
17. Klinger, R., Kolářik, C., Fluck, J., Hofmann-Apitius, M., Friedrich, C.M.: Detection of IUPAC and IUPAC-like chemical names. Bioinformatics **24**(13), i268–i276 (2008)
18. Lafferty, J., McCallum, A., Pereira, F.C.: Conditional random fields: probabilistic models for segmenting and labeling sequence data (2001)
19. Lai, T., Ji, H., Zhai, C., Tran, Q.H.: Joint biomedical entity and relation extraction with knowledge-enhanced collective inference. arXiv preprint arXiv:2105.13456 (2021)
20. Leaman, R., Gonzalez, G.: Banner: an executable survey of advances in biomedical named entity recognition. In: Biocomputing 2008, pp. 652–663. World Scientific (2008)
21. Lee, J., et al.: Biobert: a pre-trained biomedical language representation model for biomedical text mining. Bioinformatics **36**(4), 1234–1240 (2020)
22. Li, J., et al.: BioCreative V CDR task corpus: a resource for chemical disease relation extraction. Database **2016** (2016)
23. Li, X., Luo, X., Dong, C., Yang, D., Luan, B., He, Z.: Tdeer: an efficient translating decoding schema for joint extraction of entities and relations. In: Proceedings of the 2021 Conference on Empirical Methods in Natural Language Processing, pp. 8055–8064 (2021)
24. Liu, F., Chen, J., Jagannatha, A., Yu, H.: Learning for biomedical information extraction: Methodological review of recent advances. arXiv preprint arXiv:1606.07993 (2016)
25. Liu, S., Sun, Y., Li, B., Wang, W., Zhao, X.: Hamner: headword amplified multi-span distantly supervised method for domain specific named entity recognition. In: Proceedings of the AAAI Conference on Artificial Intelligence, vol. 34, pp. 8401–8408 (2020)
26. Nasar, Z., Jaffry, S.W., Malik, M.K.: Named entity recognition and relation extraction: state-of-the-art. ACM Comput. Surv. (CSUR) **54**(1), 1–39 (2021)

27. Ouyang, S., Yao, X., Wang, Y.: An overview of the text mining task for "gene-disease" association semantics. J. Med. Inform. **43**(12), 6–9 (2022)
28. Ouyang, S., Yao, X., Wang, Y.: Text mining task for "gene-disease" association semantics in chip 2022. In: Health Information Processing: 8th China Conference, CHIP 2022, Hangzhou, China, 21–23 October 2022, Revised Selected Papers. Springer, Cham (2022)
29. Peng, H., et al.: Learning from context or names? an empirical study on neural relation extraction. arXiv preprint arXiv:2010.01923 (2020)
30. Perera, N., Dehmer, M., Emmert-Streib, F.: Named entity recognition and relation detection for biomedical information extraction. Front. Cell Dev. Biol. 673 (2020)
31. Rappaport, N., et al.: Malacards: an integrated compendium for diseases and their annotation. Database **2013** (2013)
32. Rink, B., Harabagiu, S., Roberts, K.: Automatic extraction of relations between medical concepts in clinical texts. J. Am. Med. Inform. Assoc. **18**(5), 594–600 (2011)
33. Rocktäschel, T., Weidlich, M., Leser, U.: Chemspot: a hybrid system for chemical named entity recognition. Bioinformatics **28**(12), 1633–1640 (2012)
34. Safran, M., et al.: Genecards version 3: the human gene integrator. Database **2010** (2010)
35. Skreta, M., Arbabi, A., Wang, J., Brudno, M.: Training without training data: improving the generalizability of automated medical abbreviation disambiguation. In: Machine Learning for Health Workshop, pp. 233–245. PMLR (2020)
36. Song, M., Kim, W.C., Lee, D., Heo, G.E., Kang, K.Y.: PKDE4J: entity and relation extraction for public knowledge discovery. J. Biomed. Inform. **57**, 320–332 (2015)
37. Su, P., Li, G., Wu, C., Vijay-Shanker, K.: Using distant supervision to augment manually annotated data for relation extraction. PLoS ONE **14**(7), e0216913 (2019)
38. Wang, Y., Yu, B., Zhang, Y., Liu, T., Zhu, H., Sun, L.: Tplinker: single-stage joint extraction of entities and relations through token pair linking. arXiv preprint arXiv:2010.13415 (2020)
39. Wei, J., Zou, K.: EDA: easy data augmentation techniques for boosting performance on text classification tasks. arXiv preprint arXiv:1901.11196 (2019)
40. Wei, Z., Su, J., Wang, Y., Tian, Y., Chang, Y.: A novel cascade binary tagging framework for relational triple extraction. arXiv preprint arXiv:1909.03227 (2019)
41. Ye, Z.X., Ling, Z.H.: Multi-level matching and aggregation network for few-shot relation classification. arXiv preprint arXiv:1906.06678 (2019)
42. Zheng, H., et al.: PRGC: potential relation and global correspondence based joint relational triple extraction. arXiv preprint arXiv:2106.09895 (2021)
43. Zong, H., Lei, J., Li, Z.: Overview of technology evaluation dataset for medical multimodal information extraction. J. Med. Inform. **43**(12), 2–5, 12 (2022)

Biomedical Named Entity Recognition Under Low-Resource Situation

Jianfei Zhao, Xiangyu Ren(✉), Shuo Zhao, and Jinyi Li

School of Computer Science, Beijing Institute of Technology, Beijing, China
{zhaojianfei,3120210990,zhaoshuo,lijinyi}@bit.edu.cn

Abstract. Biomedical named entity recognition is Key technology for automatic processing of health medical information. However, it is labor-expensive for get enough labeled data and always facing low-resource situation. We propose a method for biomedical named entity recognition that under low-resource situation. Our work is based on the 8th China Health Information Processing Conference task-1 and ranked third among all the teams. In the final results of the test set, the precision is 38.07%, the recall is 51.04% and the F1-score is 43.61.

Keywords: Biomedical Entity · Named Entity Recognition · Low-Resource

1 Introduction

With the informationization of medical technology, more and more information data are generated which is impossible to coped manually. Thanks to prosperity of the Natural Language Processing (NLP), the automatic processing of biomedical text data is realized. Biomedical Named Entity Recognition (BioNER) is the fundamental technology and the initial step for other works, such as relation extraction [2] and semantic role labeling [1]. The purpose of the BioNER is to identify biomedical named entities such as genes, proteins, diseases and chemicals in the unstructured biomedical literature, and do structural analysis of biomedical literature base on the results of BioNER subsequently.

Recently, deep learning methods become prevalent in many research areas because they discover hidden features automatically and effectively. They have already been successfully applied to recognize biomedical named entities. The architecture of BioNER is always be divided into two module: an encoder to extract entities' features and a classifier to label entities [17]. Deep learning for end-to-end tasks requires a large amounts of data with high-quality labels, and the field of tasks also affects the performance of a model, especially in biomedical domain. Because of the difficulty of data annotation in biomedical field, several BioNER works are established under the condition of low-resource, which using data augmentation [18] or few-shot learning [19] strategy to make up for scarce annotated data and achieved great performance.

B. Tang et al. (Eds.): CHIP 2022, CCIS 1773, pp. 41–47, 2023.
https://doi.org/10.1007/978-981-99-4826-0_4

After years of development, BioNER technology tends to be mature, but its application in CHIP task-1 that *text mining task for gene-disease association semantics* [12] needs to face some unique characteristics. We have deeply analyzed the CHIP task-1, as compared to other works of BioNER, this task has the following characteristics: (1) The number of samples in the test set is much larger than that in the train set. (2) Biomedical named entities are always be unique and the ambiguity of words is rare. (3) Distribution of biomedical named entities in text data is sparse and there is almost no nested problem. Considering the above characteristics of CHIP task-1, we propose a method for BioNER under low-resource situation.

The following content will be organize as follows: Sect. 2 will introduce some related works, Sect. 3 will introduce our method in detail, Sect. 4 will analysis our method and display experiment results, Sect. 5 will conclude our work.

2 Related Works

The NER task always be modeled as sequence labeling task that give a text $x_1, x_2, \cdots x_N$ and get a sequence of labels $y_1, y_2 \cdots y_N$, where y_i denotes whether the token x_i is entity or the type of entity and N denotes length of sequence. The most common annotation scheme for NER is BIO tagging, where B means the beginning token of entity, I for the inside tokens and O for the tokens outside entities. In this way, the number of labels becomes $2M + 1$ from M. Conditional Random Field (CRF) [3] is always be used because of the strong logicality that the label-I always follows the label-B in BIO tagging.

There are many works use CRF behind an encoder to classify tokens in input sequence [4–6]. The main difference between those works is encoder. LSTM is the most used network act as encoder's backbone, and based on that appears Bi-LSTM with bidirecational context and Attn-LSTM with attention mechanism. Great success of Pre-trained model has led to strong textual representation, especially BioBERT [7], a bidirectional Transformer Encoder trained by large-scale Biomedical text data achieved excellent results in BioNER task. There have some works based on BioBERT and made progress. Tong et al. [8] enrich granularities of contextual features by tag-level and sentence-level subtasks. Cong et al. [9] formalized NER task as machine reading comprehension framework that extracting answer blocks from context based on entity question. In addition to improving the encoder, there are also have work adapt classifier. Wei et al. [20] masks illegal transitions during CRF training, eliminating illegal outcomes in a principled way. Such end-to-end architecture of encoder and classifier is easy to train, simple and efficient, but easy to overfit without sufficient training data.

Few-shot learning is a typical strategy to deal with low-resource problem. Few-shot learning methods [13] always build support set and label samples via contrasting similarity between support sample and test sample. Additionally, some works introduce meta-learning [16], which train a prototype representation for each labels and then select prototype for each test sample by distance between embeddings. These methods effectively alleviate the problem of low resources.

However, for CHIP task-1, there are not enough unlabeled data for representation learning because of its specific field.

3 Methods

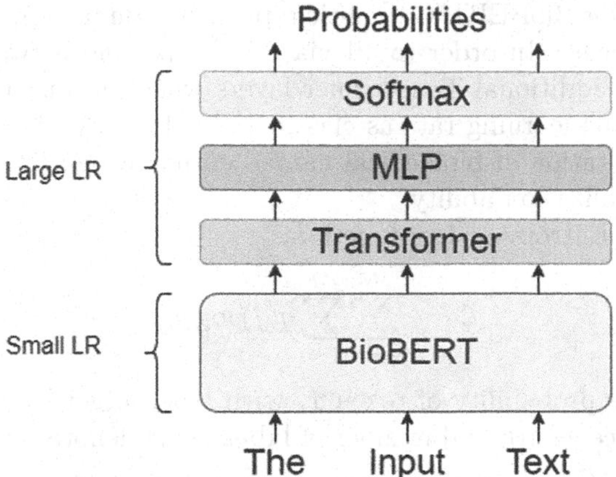

Fig. 1. The Model have additional Transformer layers on top of BioBERT, and use MLP to project token representation to label probabilities. The BioBERT is Pre-trained and use small learning rate. The others is initiated and use large learning rate.

Considering the specific situation of CHIP task-1, that low-resource, specific named entities and sparse labels, we propose our BioNER method based on the idea that using transfer learning of pre-training biomedical model and retaining its generalization.

The architecture of our model is shown in Fig. 1 We use BioBERT as our encoder to get representation of each token in text and do classification task over that. Considering the unique of word in biomedical named entity phrase and sparse of distribution, we abandon BIO tagging and classify word to entity type directly, because there is almost no entity nesting problem and task complexity is reduced in some extent because of less label types. Specifically, during training we use named entity type as label to annotate all tokens in an entity. At inference, the label of the word depend on the first token in it. Comparing to the BIO tagging, there is less logicality between labels in our annotation method, so we use a Multi-Layer Perceptron (MLP) classifier to label tokens rather than CRF. MLP is a typical classifier with a fully connected hidden layer between the output layer and the input layer, and converts the output of the hidden layer through activation function. MLP can convert hidden state of token into probability distribution of labels, and wildly used in many classification task, such as text classification [14] and named entity recognition [15] We will show the difference between MLP and CRF by experiment in Sect. 4.

Because of the low-resource situation, training model directly tend to be overfitting, and lost generalization of the pre-trained model. We use different learning rate between pre-trained parameters and initialized parameters to retain the background knowledge that the model learned during the pre-training. BioBERT use smaller learning rate finetune and the classifier use larger, both using separate optimizer.

Different learning rate also arise a new problem that smaller learning rate makes it difficult for BioBERT's semantic representation to adapt to downstream task in fewer epoches. In order to alleviate incompatible between encoder and classifier, we add additional Transformer layers with initialized before classifier which has the same learning rate as classifier. In this way, the model can learn semantic representation of biomedical named entity recognition task while preserving the generalization ability.

We use Cross-Entropy as loss function:

$$\mathcal{L} = -\sum_{i=0}^{N}\sum_{j=0}^{M} q(j)\log p_{ij} \tag{1}$$

where p_{ij} denotes probability of token x_i with label y_i get by classifier, N and M denote sequence length and number of labels, $q(j)$ denotes labelsmoothing to alleviate overfitting:

$$\begin{cases} q(j) = 1 - \beta & \text{if } j = l_i \\ q(j) = \beta/(M-1) & \text{if } j \neq l_i \end{cases} \tag{2}$$

4 Experiment

4.1 Dataset

The data is from Active Gene Annotation Corpus (AGAC) [11], this corpus is mainly used to explore the gene-disease association mechanism caused by mutations. The train set is public and contains 250 samples with 12 label types, the test set is secret and have 2000 samples. We divide public train set into train set with 200 samples and validate set with 50 samples.

4.2 Experiment Setting

We use *dmis-lab/biobert-base-cased-v1.2* as our encoder and add additional two layers Transformer with same dimension as BioBERT on top of it. We use AdamW [10] as optimizer, the learning rate of MLP and Transformers is $2e-3$ and BioBERT is $3e-5$. The dimension of hidden layer in MLP is 4096 and use GELU as active function. We train model 150 epoches on train set and select the checkpoint with best F1-score on the validate set.

In order to demonstrate effective of each component, we build four variants to do ablation study: *CRF*, use BioBERT encode text and use CRF as classifier. *MLP*, use BioBERT encode text and use MLP as classifier. MLP_{sep_rl}, BioBERT and MLP use separate optimizer with different learning rate. $Trans{+}MLP_{sep\_rl}$, add additional Transformer layers before MLP.

Table 1. Ablation study results, **P** denotes precision score, **R** denotes recall score, **F1** denotes F1-score

Model	P	R	F1
Validate Set			
CRF	77.5	79.5	78.5
MLP	76.9	83.9	80.3
MLP_{sep_rl}	78.8	83.9	81.3
$Trans{+}MLP_{sep\_rl}$	**79.9**	**85.9**	**82.8**
Test set			
$Trans{+}MLP_{sep\_rl}$	38.07	51.04	43.61

4.3 Main Results

The main results is shown in Table 1. Using F1-score as criterion, we can see MLP classifier, separate learning rate and additional Transformer layers are all effective. We also record the F1-score on validate set during the model training, the fluctuation of F1-score is shown in Fig. 2. we calculate the variance of F1-scores to reflect generalization ability, we can see that $Trans{+}MLP_{sep\_rl}$ has the lowest variance and it demonstrate our method can effectively mitigate overfitting. Finally, we use $Trans{+}MLP_{sep\_rl}$ as our model to generate test set results and submit to CHIP platform. The Detailed evaluation results of the test set shown in Table 2.

Table 2. Detailed results of the test set.

Type	Gene	Reg	Dise	Var	PosReg	Ptn	CPA	NegReg	MPA	Inter	Enzyme	Pth
P	36.76	38.24	44.06	31.79	47.76	31.68	39.74	33.79	52.46	42.86	41.18	29.49
R	52.03	63.76	39.53	62.92	53.85	41.67	62.57	52.01	51.86	52.83	51.11	50.30
F1	43.08	47.80	46.97	35.24	54.30	39.89	40.68	40.97	57.07	47.33	46.28	37.40

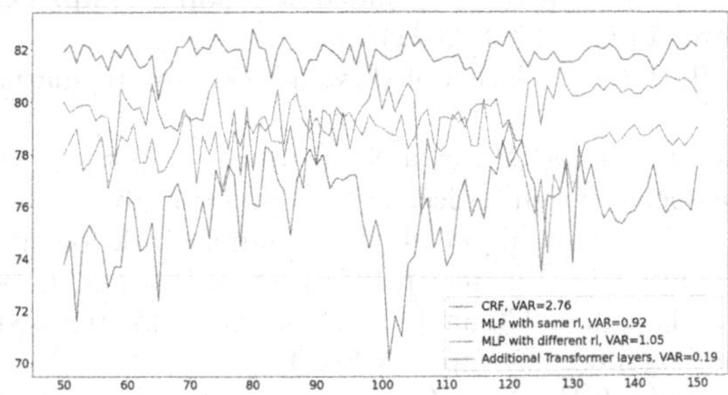

Fig. 2. The F1-scores on validate set during the model training.

5 Conclusion

We propose a named biomedical entity recognition method for low-resource situation based on characteristics of 8th CHIP task-1. Specifically, we use the BioBERT as backbone and add additional two Transformer layers to alleviate incompatible semantic representation between pre-training and downstream task caused by small learning rate. Because of the sparse and unique of biomedical named entities, We abandon classical BIO tagging scheme and use MLP to classify tokens label type to reduce complexity of task. In the 8th CHIP task-1 evaluation, we ranked third. In the future work, we will further explore the potential of the pre-training model to better fit low-resource situation.

References

1. Jiang, B., Lan, Y.: Research on semantic role labeling method. ChinaCom. 252–258 (2018)
2. Patel, R., Tanwani, S., Patidar, C.: Relation extraction between medical entities using deep learning approach. Informatica (Slovenia). **45**(3) (2021)
3. Lafferty, J.D., McCallum, A., Pereira, F.C.N.: Conditional random fields: probabilistic models for segmenting and labeling sequence data. In: ICML 2001, pp. 282–289 (2001)
4. Symeonidou, A., Sazonau, V., Groth, P.: Transfer learning for biomedical named entity recognition with BioBERT. In: SEMANTiCS (Posters & Demos) (2019)
5. Luo, L.: An attention-based BiLSTM-CRF approach to document-level chemical named entity recognition. Bioinformatics **34**(8), 1381–1388 (2018)
6. Habibi, M., Weber, L., Neves, M.L., Wiegandt, D.L., Leser, U.: Deep learning with word embeddings improves biomedical named entity recognition. Bioinformatics **33**(14), i37–i48 (2017)
7. Lee, J., et al.: BioBERT: a pre-trained biomedical language representation model for biomedical text mining. Bioinformatics **36**(4), 1234–1240 (2020)
8. Tong, Y., Chen, Y., Shi, X.: A multi-task approach for improving biomedical named entity recognition by incorporating multi-granularity information. In: Findings of the Association for Computational Linguistics: ACL-IJCNLP 2021, pp. 4804–4813. Association for Computational Linguistics, Online (2021)
9. Sun, C., Yang, Z., Wang, L., Zhang, Y., Lin, H., Wang, J.: Biomedical named entity recognition using BERT in the machine reading comprehension framework. J. Biomed. Inform. **118**, 103799 (2021)
10. Loshchilov, I., Hutter, F.: Decoupled weight decay regularization. In: ICLR (Poster) (2019)
11. Ouyang, S., Yao, X., Wang, Y., et al.: An overview of the text mining task for "gene-disease" association semantics. J. Med. Inform. **43**(12), 6–9 (2022)
12. Ouyang, S., Yao, X., Wang, Y., et al.: Text mining task for "gene-disease" association semantics in CHIP. In: Health Information Processing: 8th China Conference, CHIP 2022, Hangzhou, China, October 21–23, 2022, Revised Selected Papers. Springer Nature Singapore, Singapore (2022)
13. Li, X., Sun, Z., Xue, J.-H., Ma, Z.: A concise review of recent few-shot meta-learning methods. Neurocomputing **456**, 463–468 (2021)

14. Zhang, Y., Yu, X., Cui, Z., Wu, S., Wen, Z., Wang, L.: Every document owns its structure: inductive text classification via graph neural networks. In: ACL 2020, pp. 334–339 (2020)
15. Nguyen, N., Miwa, M.: Span-based named entity recognition by generating and compressing information. In: EACL, Sophia Ananiadou, pp. 1976–1988 (2023)
16. Bin, J., et al.: Few-shot named entity recognition with entity-level prototypical network enhanced by dispersedly distributed prototypes. In: COLING 2022, pp. 1842–1854 (2022)
17. Song, B., Li, F., Liu, Y., Zeng, X.: Deep learning methods for biomedical named entity recognition: a survey and qualitative comparison. Brief. Bioinform. **22**(6) (2021)
18. Phan, U., Nguyen, N.: Simple semantic-based data augmentation for named entity recognition in biomedical texts. In: BioNLP@ACL 2022, pp. 123–129 (2022)
19. Kosprdic, M., Prodanovic, N., Ljajic, A., Basaragin, B., Milosevic, N.: A transformer-based method for zero and few-shot biomedical named entity recognition. CoRR abs/2305.04928 (2023)
20. Wei, T., Qi, J., He, S.: Masked conditional random fields for sequence labeling. In: NAACL-HLT, pp. 2024–2035. Songtao Sun (2021)

Medical Causal Entity and Relation Extraction

CHIP2022 Shared Task Overview: Medical Causal Entity Relationship Extraction

Zihao Li[1], Mosha Chen[1(✉)], Kangping Yin[1], Yixuan Tong[1], Chuanqi Tan[1], Zhenzhen Lang[1], and Buzhou Tang[2,3]

[1] Alibaba Group, Hangzhou310000, Zhejiang, China
chenmosha.cms@alibaba-inc.com

[2] Harbin Institute of Technology (Shenzhen), Shenzhen 518055, Guangdong, China

[3] Pengcheng Laboratory, Shenzhen 518055, Guangdong, China

Abstract. Modern medicine emphasizes interpretability and requires doctors to give reasonable, well-founded and convincing diagnostic results when diagnosing patients. Therefore, there are a large number of causal correlations in medical concepts such as symptoms, diagnosis and treatment in the text of the results of the inquiry. Explanation of relationships, and mining these relationships from text is of great help in improving the accuracy and interpretability of medical search results. Based on this, this paper constructs a new medical causality extraction dataset CMedCausal (**C**hinese **Med**ical **Causal** dataset) and it is used in the CHIP2022 shared task, which defines three key types of medical causal relationships: causal relationship, conditional relationship, and hypothetical relationship. It consists of 9,153 medical texts with a total of 79,244 entity relationships annotated. Participants need to correctly label these correct reasoning relationships and corresponding subject-object entities. A total of 49 teams submitted results for the preliminary round with the highest Macro-F1 value of 0.4510. A total of 25 teams submitted results for final round with the highest Macro-F1 value of 0.4416.

Keywords: causal relationship · relation extraction · interpretability

1 Introduction

Online medical QA texts on the Internet contain a large number of medical-related concepts [1,2]. How to leverage natural language processing and deep learning technology to obtain relevant medical knowledge has received widespread attention in recent years. However, the complexity and diversity of medical concepts and the privacy of medical data have posed great challenges for related research.

The entity and relationship extraction technology in the medical field can identify medical concepts and the interrelationships between concepts, and applying this knowledge to the medical knowledge graph can help effectively

B. Tang et al. (Eds.): CHIP 2022, CCIS 1773, pp. 51–56, 2023.
https://doi.org/10.1007/978-981-99-4826-0_5

improve the interpretability of the medical graph. It is expensive to manually construct these graphs. In order to obtain more and more accurate relational knowledge, it is necessary to automatically obtain this knowledge through entity-relationship joint extraction technology [3,4].

2 Related Work

In recent years, academic organizations such as the international biological and clinical informatics integrated research project i2b2 (Informatics for Integrating Biology and the Bedside) and the China Health Information Processing Conference CHIP (China Health Information Processing Conference) have actively advocated mining useful information from medical data. They organized a series of shared tasks, which have gained wide influence in the research community and played an important role in the field of medical information processing.

At present, researchers have proposed a number of causality extraction datasets, such as Mariko [5] et al. proposed FinCausal based on the financial field, and Tan [6] et al. proposed the causal relationship extraction task based on the news field. In the medical field, the BioCreativeV community proposed the task of automatically extracting causal entities from biomedical literature and representing them with related sentences [7]. However, Chinese datasets are still relatively scarce. Therefore, this paper makes full use of medical search engines and medical answer texts from online consultations to construct the first Chinese medical causality extraction data CMedCausal, and release the "Medical Causal Entity Relationship Extraction" shared task on the CHIP2022 conference [8]. Researchers can use CMedCausal [9] to conduct research for medical causality mining and causal explanation network construction, so as to improve the interpretability of medical consultation results.

3 Dataset

3.1 Task Definition

The CMedCausal is derived from the youlai website[1]. Since it is from public online consultation data, few privacy information is involved, so no special desensitization is required. The filtered text contains a total of 9,153 paragraphs of text with an average length of 265 characters.

The dataset needs to label the medical concept mention and the relationship between the medical concept mention. A medical concept mention refers to a continuous text span that can be used as an independent semantic unit. The relationship between medical concept mentions includes the following three types:

Causal Relation refers to a certain cause that directly leads to a certain result. For example: "人体的胃肠道功能紊乱，导致患者吸收能力变差", In this

[1] https://m.youlai.cn.

example "胃肠道功能紊乱" is a direct cause of "吸收能力变差", "吸收能力变差" is a direct result of "胃肠道功能紊乱".

Conditional Relationship refers to some specific conditions in medical concept fragments, which are used to modify specific causal relationships. For example: "对阿莫西林过敏的患者不可以使用，服用阿莫西林可能会引起皮疹、药物热和哮喘等过敏反应，因此使用前一定要做青霉素皮试试验", "对阿莫西林过敏" in this example is the condition for "服用阿莫西林" to cause "皮疹".

Hypernym Relationship refers to the concept of a broad general term containing a specific and special concept. For example: "阿尔茨海默症是一种精神类疾病", In this example "精神类疾病" includes the specific mention "阿尔茨海默症".

3.2 Data Annotation

The annotation was completed by 8 medical undergraduates led by 1 medical expert and 1 AI algorithm expert based on Alibaba Quark's internal labeling tool. It took 1.5 months before and after, and the total cost was 54,000 RMB. The number of labeled causal relationships, conditional relationships, and hyponymy relationships are 70,564, 3,819, and 4,861, respectively, and the proportional distribution of the three types of relationships is 18.5:1:1.3. The labeling process is shown in Fig. 1. Table 1 shows the details of the train, dev and test set.

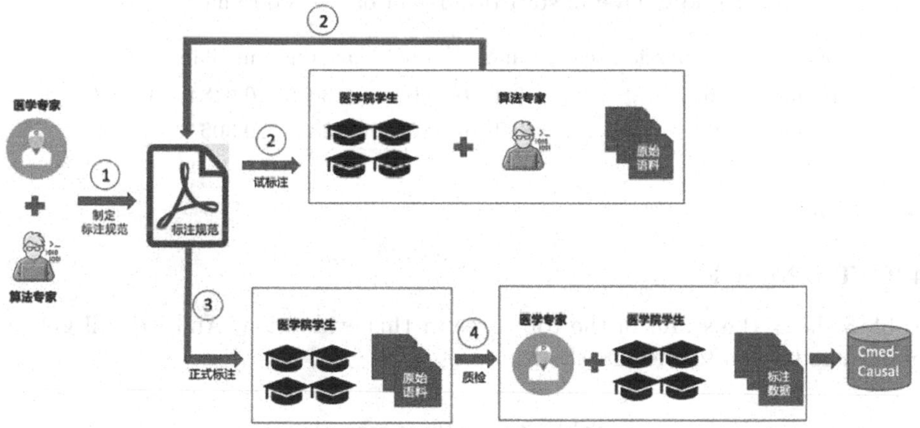

Fig. 1. Schematic diagram of CMedCausal labeling process

Table 1. Statistics of the labeled data

split	number of sample	average character length	causal	conditional	hypenym	proportion
train set	7355	265	55457	3042	3914	18.23:1:1.29
dev set	915	271	7096	375	469	18.92:1:1.25
test set	916	256	8011	402	478	19.92:1:1.19

3.3 Evaluation Metric

This task uses precision (P), recall (R) and F1 score (F-Measure, F1) as evaluation metrics. Considering that the proportions of the three types of relationships are quite different, this task uses Macro-F1 serves as the final evaluation criterion.

Specific definition, assuming that there are n categories, C_1, C_i,C_n, the calculation formula is as follows: Let the number of samples correctly predicted as category C_i be $T_p(i)$, the number of samples predicted as C_i is T_i, and the real The number of samples of C_i is P_i.

$$Precision_i = \frac{T_{p(i)}}{T_i}$$
$$Recall_i = \frac{T_{p(i)}}{P_i}$$
$$Macro - F1 = \frac{1}{n}\sum_{i=1}^{n}\frac{2*Precision_i*Recall_i}{Precision_i+Recall_i}$$

4 Submission Result

4.1 Overall Statistics

The shared task is divided into two phases: the preliminary round(Round A) and the final round(Round B). The statistical result was shown in Table 2.

Table 2. Overall statistical result of the two rounds

phase	submission teams	max	min	average	median	std
Round A	49	0.4510	0.0790	0.3049	0.3184	0.1177
Round B	25	0.4416	0.0859	0.3325	0.3064	0.1188

4.2 Top Models

Table 3 shows the scores of the top three in this evaluation. And we will give a brief introduction to their methods.

Table 3. Top three scores

ranking	organization	Marco-F1
1st	Pacific Insurance Technology	0.4416
2nd	Beijing Health Home Technology	0.4355
3th	Winning Health Technology Group	0.4323

The first team splits the task into two subtasks: entity recognition and relationship classification. In the entity recognition stage, the token-pair matrix is used to identify the start and end positions of entities to identify entities in sentences. In the relationship classification stage, the contestants use the PL-Marker method [10] to insert identifiers before and after the subject in the sentence, and at the same time insert the corresponding object identifier after the sentence to share the same position id with the object. The output score of the object identifier is used for the relationship classification.

The second team regards the task as a joint extraction of entities and relationships. First, the feature matrix is obtained through biaffine attention calculation, and then the corresponding relation triplet is obtained through joint extraction. In particular, the contestant split the conditional relations of three entities into three corresponding triplets.

The third team uses the token-pair feature matrix to extract common causality and hypernym triplet, and uses machine reading comprehension(MRC) mechanism to extract nested conditional relationships. The contestant used filtering partitions to alleviate the problem of overlapping relationships. In addition, they designed an undersampling contrastive learning method to improve the model's ability to extract conditional relationships.

5 Conclusion

This paper introduces the construction of the first Chinese medical causal dataset CMedCausal and the models and performance of the top contestants during the CHIP2022 shared task. The dataset contains the three most common types of relationships in medical causal inference: causal relationships, conditional relationships, and hypernym relationships. Researchers can use CMedCausal for further study.

References

1. Raja, U., Mitchell, T., Day, T., et al.: Text mining in healthcare. applications and opportunities. J. Healthcare Inf. Manage. JHIM. **22**(3), 52–56 (2008)
2. Esteva, A., Robicquet, A., Ramsundar, B., et al.: A guide to deep learning in healthcare. Nat. Med. **25**, 24–29 (2019)
3. Uzuner, Ö., South, B.R., Shen, S., et al.: 2010 i2b2/va challenge on concepts, assertions, and relations in clinical text. J. Am. Med. Inform. Assoc. **18**(5), 552–556 (2011)
4. Chang, D., Chen, M., Liu, C., et al.: DiaKG: an annotated diabetes dataset for medical knowledge graph construction. arXiv preprint arXiv:2105.15033 (2021)
5. Dominique, M., Labidurie, E., Ozturk, Y., et al.: Data Processing and Annotation Schemes for FinCausal Shared Task. arXiv preprint arXiv:2012.02498 (2020)
6. Tan, F.A., Hürriyetoğlu, A., Caselli, T., et al.: The Causal News Corpus: Annotating Causal Relations in Event Sentences from News. arXiv preprint arXiv:2204.11714 (2022)
7. 刘苏文, 邵一帆, 钱龙华, 等. 基于联合学习的生物医学因果关系抽取 [J]. 中文信息学报 , 2020, 34(4):60–68

8. Zong, H., Lei, J., Li, Z., et al.: Overview of technology evaluation dataset for medical multimodal information extraction. J. Med. Inform. **43**(12), 2–5+22 (2022)
9. Li, Z., Chen, M., Ma, Z., et al.: CMedCausal: Chinese medical causal relationship extraction dataset. J. Med. Inform. **43**(12), 23–27+31 (2022)
10. Ye, D., Lin, Y., Li, P., et al.: Packed levitated marker for entity and relation extraction. arXiv preprint arXiv:2109.06067 (2021)

Domain Robust Pipeline for Medical Causal Entity and Relation Extraction Task

Tao Liang, Shengjun Yuan(✉), Pengfei Zhou, Hangcong Fu, and Huizhe Wu

Pacific Insurance Technology Co., Ltd., Shanghai 200010, China
yuanshengjun@cpic.com.cn

Abstract. Medical entity and relation extraction is an essential task for medical knowledge graph, which can provide explanatory answers for medical search engine. Recently, PL-Marker, a deep learning based pipeline, has been proposed, which follows a similar NER&ER paradigm. In this method, medical entities are first identified by a NER model, and then they are combined by pairs to feed into a ER model to learn the causal relation among the medical entities. In this way, the pipeline cannot handle the complex entity relationships contained by CMedCausal due to its own defects, such as exposure bias and lack of relevance between entities and relationships. In this paper, we propose a novel pipeline: Domain Robust Pipeline (DRP) which tackles these challenges by introducing noisy entities to solve the exposure bias, adding KL loss to learn from samples with noisy labels, applying multitask learning to escape semantic traps and re-targeting the relationships to increase the robustness of the pipeline.

Keywords: Medical entity extraction · Medical causal relation determination · Domain robust pipeline

1 Introduction

1.1 Background

There are a large number of causal correlations in medical concepts such as symptoms, diagnosis and treatment in the text of the results of the inquiry. Based on this, CMedCausal (Chinese Medical Causal Relations Extraction Dataset) [1] defines three types of medical causal explanation and reasoning relationships: causal relationship, conditional relationship, and hypothetical relationship. It consists of 9,153 medical texts with a total of 79,244 entity relationships annotated. In a competition "Medical Causal Entity Relationship Extraction" held by CHIP (China Health Information Processing Conference[1]), the training dataset

[1] CHIP is an annual conference aiming to explore the mystery of life, improve the quality of health, and develop the level of medical treatment with the help of information processing technologies. http://www.cips-chip.org.cn/.

B. Tang et al. (Eds.): CHIP 2022, CCIS 1773, pp. 57–65, 2023.
https://doi.org/10.1007/978-981-99-4826-0_6

contains 1000 medical texts with imbalanced distribution of the entity relationships. Most of the relationships are a kind of one-to-many SEO (Single Entity Overlap) relation. Therefore, PL-Marker (Packed Levitated Marker) [2], which is supposed to have a good performance on one-to-many SEO relationship extraction task, is selected as the backbone by us.

1.2 Data Description

The performance of a simple application of PL-Marker on CMedCausal doesn't meet our expectations. After we have a deep insight of CMedCausal, we find five problems which could not be handled by the standard pipeline.

Semantic Traps. Since we divide the medical causal entity and relation extraction task into two steps, some semantic traps have been caused by the pipeline structure as shown below.

- "Taking **amoxicillin** may cause **anaphylaxis** like skin rash, drug fever and asthma."
- "Amoxicillin has a certain auxiliary effect in the treatment of reversible pulpitis, but it is generally not used."

According to the marking criteria, "amoxicillin" is marked as a medical entity in the first sentence but in the second sentence is not. However, a simple NER model[2] (Named Entity Recognizer) can not find the difference between these two sentences. In most cases, it wrongly predicts "amoxicillin" as a medical entity in the second sentence, which will bring some mistakes in the relation extraction step.

Defective Data. During the analysis of the bad cases in our pipeline, we find that the similar medical entities have different boundaries in different sentences.

- "For patients with wind-cold cold, fever will not be particularly serious, and patients will **have obvious fear of cold and cold**."
- "It is the manifestation of conjunctival calculus, which is a common disease in ophthalmology. Patients will have **obvious strange body sensation**."

Here we can see that "have" is labeled as a part of the entity in the first sentence but in the second sentence is not. A regular pattern for the boundaries of the spans of words is absent. Moreover, some entity relationships are annotated with wrong labels.

[2] We use Bert as a pre-trained language model for the entity extraction task.

Exposure Bias. Exposure bias is a common problem of the pipeline for the entity and relation extraction task. In training process, since we have the true medical entities for a given sentence, the ER (Entity Relationship) model has a dataset without errors. But in the serving process, the inputs of the ER model, which are the outputs of the NER model, usually deviate the true entities as the following.

- "Taking amoxicillin may cause **anaphylaxis** like **skin rash**, **drug fever** and **asthma** [ground truth]."
- "Taking amoxicillin may cause **anaphylaxis** like **skin rash**, **drug fever and asthma** [outputs of the NER model]."

Single Entity Overlap. In the whole dataset, we find that all the entity relationships can be classed as Single Entity Overlap (SEO), which means that there is only one entity repeated in different relationships of one text, either the subject or the object. And SEO can also be divided into two types: one-to-many relationships and many-to-one relationships.

- "Taking amoxicillin may cause **anaphylaxis** like **skin rash**, **drug fever** and **asthma**."
- "**Cerebral infarction** can be caused by many reasons. The most common reason is **atherosclerosis**, followed by **hyperlipemia**, **hyperglycemia**, **severe hypotension** and **the shedding of various emboli**."

In the first sentence, the subject "amoxicillin" has causal relationships with many objects such as "skin rash", "drug fever" and "asthma". It can be classified as one-to-many relationship. While in the second sentence, one object "cerebral infarction" is caused by multiple subjects like "atherosclerosis", "hyperlipemia", "hyperglycemia", "severe hypotension" and "the shedding of various emboli". It can be categorized as many-to-one relationship.

Three-Element Relationship. Differing from the other two entity relationships, conditional relationship contains three elements: condition, cause and result.

- "If you are **pregnant**, and **have abdominal pain** or **vaginal bleeding**, it can be regarded as **a threatened abortion**."

In this medical text, with "pregnant" as the condition, "have abdominal pain" and "vaginal bleeding" are the reasons of "a threatened abortion". Thus, we need a novel structure of model to handle this challenge, because a standard PL-Marker can only predict a two-element relationship.

2 Domain Robust Pipeline

Different from other entity relationships, medical causal relationships are mainly composed of one-to-many relationships. Single-stage joint extraction model such as TP-Linker (Token-Pair Linker) [3] cannot effectively extract the information between multiple objects. Effective approaches are required to extract the relationships between one subject and multiple objects. Subject-oriented packing for span pairs [2] is a novel method which can build a representation of the span pairs as shown in Fig. 1. Making use of this method is critical for medical causal relation extraction. Moreover, TP-Linker can also serve as a NER model in the first step of the PL-Marker pipeline[3].

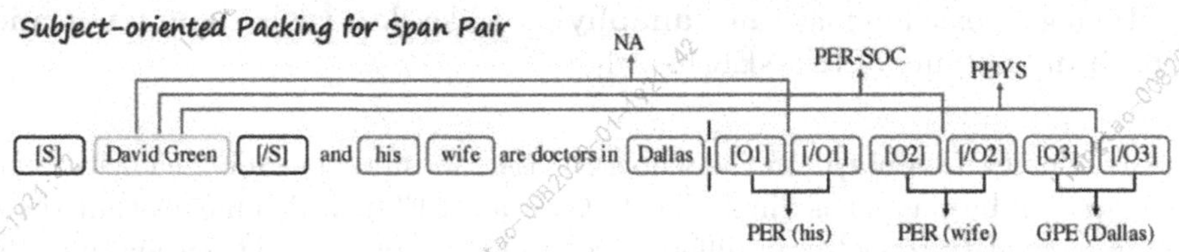

Fig. 1. Subject-oriented packing for the span pairs packs objects with the same subject.

2.1 Base Model (TP-Linker)

Since TP-Linker achieved SOTA (State-of-the-art) performance on WebNLG[4] and NYT[5], we refer to the TP-Linker as our base model. It consists of several important parts:

Token-Pair Tagging. For the convenience to illustrate, we use one matrix to show all the tags in Fig. 2. This tagging matrix contains three kinds of span pairs: SH-to-OH (subject head to object head), ST-to-OT (subject tail to object tail) and EH-to-ET (entity head to entity tail). Furthermore, to alleviate the sparsity of the matrix, TP-Linker maps all tag 1 in the lower triangular region to tag 2 in the upper triangular region, and then drops the lower triangular region [3]. After doing this, it is not a complete matrix anymore like Fig. 2.

Handshaking Tagger. TP-Linker utilizes a unified architecture for EH-to-ET, SH-to-OH and ST-to-OT tagging. Given a token pair (w_i and w_j), it encodes the two tokens, concatenates the two token representations as $h_{i,j}$ and predicts the link label of token pair (w_i, w_j) by following the equations below.

$$h_{i,j} = tanh(W_h \cdot [Encode(w_i); Encode(w_j)] + b_h), \ where \ j > i \tag{1}$$

[3] A PL-Marker pipeline usually consists of two serial models: a NER model and a ER model.

[4] https://synalp.gitlabpages.inria.fr/webnlg-challenge.

[5] https://open.nytimes.com/data/home.

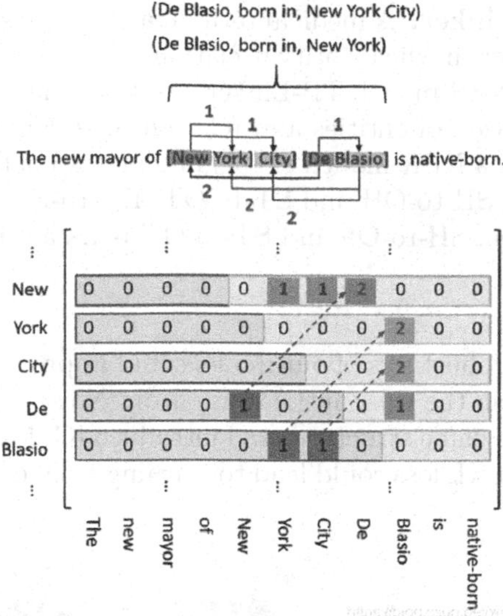

Fig. 2. A tagging matrix [3].

$$P(y_{i,j}) = Softmax(W_o \cdot h_{i,j} + b_o), \tag{2}$$

$$link(w_i, w_j) = \arg\max_l P(y_{i,j} = l), \tag{3}$$

where $P(y_{i,j} = l)$ represents the probability of identifying the link of (w_i, w_j) as l.

Global Pointer and Multi-Label Classification Loss [5] The handshaking tagging mechanism is complicated and mediocre on imbalanced dataset. Therefore, we introduce global pointer and multi-label classification loss proposed in GP-Linker (Global-Pointer Based Linker) [6]. Instead of calculating the $P_{i,j}$ of each token pair in a sentence like Eq. 2, global pointer takes use of scaled dot-product to get a probability matrix and then uses multi-label classification loss to alleviate the problem of unbalanced distribution.

$$s_\alpha(i,j) = (W_{\alpha,i} \cdot Encode(w_i) + b_{\alpha,i})^T (W_{\alpha,j} \cdot Encode(w_j) + b_{\alpha,j}), \tag{4}$$

where α means the type of the task.

2.2 Structure of Pipeline

In order to meet the challenges mentioned in data description part, we modify the standard PL-Marker by using TP-Linker as the NER model to escape the semantic traps and introducing KL loss to learn from defective data with noisy labels.

NER Model with TP-Linker. A medical term in a sentence should be part of a relationship first, then be a medical entity. Relation extraction task is supposed to be introduced into the NER model. TP-Linker has its particular advantages in a single-stage joint extraction of entities and relationships, which could provide information of relations in a NER model. A tagging matrix contains three kinds of token pairs: EH-to-ET, SH-to-OH and ST-to-OT. EH-to-ET pairs are inputs for name entity recognition, SH-to-Oh and ST-to-OT pairs are inputs for entity relation classification.

KL Loss. Increasing the robustness of our model could improve its performance on the dirty data. Referring the work in Learning from Noisy Labels [4], we initialize two models with the same structure, and introduce KL loss while training. Noisy samples having high KL loss could lead to learning from each other instead of overfitting (Fig. 3).

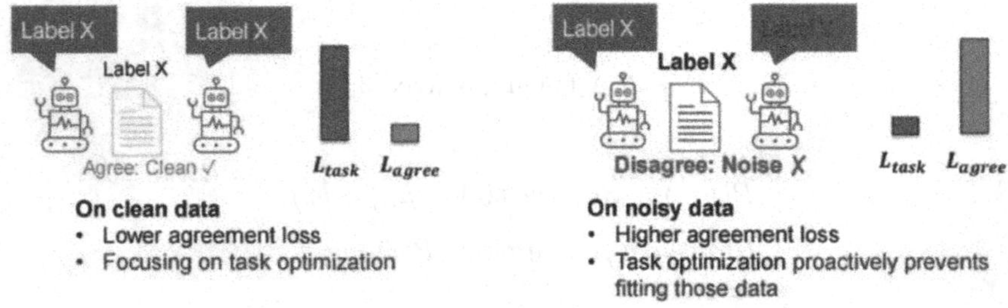

Fig. 3. We train two models synchronously and introduce KL loss to restrict the damage of noisy data.

2.3 Training Techniques

In the pipeline of medical entity and relation extraction, exposure bias and domain adaption are two great challenges. Practically, the structure of pipeline leads to training-serving-inconsistency problem, and ER model can only predict two-element relationships. In this section, we introduce two important techniques which are proven to be helpful in practice.

Introducing Noisy Data. To fix the exposure bias problem, we take a try of two ways to introduce noisy data. One is directly using the output entities of the NER model as the input of the ER model. The other is merging the predicted entities with the true entities if the predicted entities appear in the results of the NER model. According to the AB tests, we find that the second method is a better way to fix the problem.

Relationship Re-targeting. PL-Marker only supports one-to-many and two-element relationships. However, CMedCausal contains many-to-one and three-element relationships. We design a compatible pipeline by re-targeting the many-to-one and three-element relationships. To turn the many-to-one relationship into one-to-many relationship, we add a new "causative relationship"[6]. We replace the original subjects with the single object and vice versa. Similarly, we break a conditional relationship into two separate relationships: "condition-cause relationship" and common causal relationship. As a conclusion, we add two new entity relationships by relationship re-targeting to make the pipeline be compatible with the two special relationships.

3 Experiments

In this section, we present our experiments in detail, including datasets, evaluation metrics, experimental setup, model comparison and the corresponding analysis. Experiments on CMedCausal demonstrate the effectiveness of proposed approach which outperforms state-of-the-art methods on the medical causal entity and relation extraction task.

3.1 Dataset and Experimental Setup

Dataset. CMedCausal dataset contains three kinds of relationships with high unbalanced distribution. Causal relationships account for almost ninety percent. Since the average sentence length is 265, we truncate the length of input texts combined with flags to 512 characters. The statistics of the dataset is shown in Table 1.

Table 1. The statistics of CMedCausal.

Sample Size	Character Size	Average Sentence Length	Causal	Conditional	Hypothetical
7355	248761	265	55457	3042	3914

Experimental Setup. We choose TP-Linker as our base model, and PL-Marker with a TP-Linker as the backbone. First, we use a single TP-Linker for both entities recognition and relation classification tasks. Second, we only use TP-Linker as a NER model with a 3-head mechanism, and combine a ER model after the TP-Linker as our backbone. Next, we separately implement all the training techniques and structure modifications on the backbone to verify the effectiveness. Specifically, KL Loss is only applied on the ER model with two

[6] It means that the result is considered as a subject and the reason is considered as an object.

expert models. Finally, we integrate all these training techniques on the same pipeline. For all models, we use Adam [8] as the optimizer without weight decay, in which learning rate is 0.00001. The epoch number is set as 20 for both NER and ER models. We use RoBerta-Large [9] as the encoder with 512 as the length of the input texts.

3.2 Metrics

In the entity and relation extraction task as a multi-label classification task, Macro-F1 score is a widely used metric [7]. It takes consideration of both precision and recall by classifying all the identified entities. It is calculated as follows:

$$P_i = \frac{number\ of\ truly\ predicted\ samples\ for\ category\ i}{number\ of\ samples\ predicted\ as\ category\ i} \tag{5}$$

$$R_i = \frac{number\ of\ truly\ predicted\ samples\ for\ category\ i}{number\ of\ real\ samples\ for\ category\ i} \tag{6}$$

$$Macro - F1 = \frac{1}{n}\sum_{i=1}^{n} = \frac{2P_iR_i}{P_i + R_i}, \tag{7}$$

where a sample is considered as truly predicted only when both entities and relationships are truly predicted.

3.3 Performance of Pipeline

Table 2 shows the results on validation dataset. All experiments are repeated 5 times and averaged results are reported. Obviously, all the technical methods could significantly improve the performance of the pipeline. PL-Marker with a TP-Linker as the NER model [10] could be considered as the base of the mechanism, and it demonstrates the feasibility of the two-step pipeline.

Table 2. Best F1-scores of base model and backbone with different technical methods. All the other lines calculate Improvement by comparing with the first line.

Technical Method	F1-score	Improvement
TP-Linker	0.3634	0.0%
Pipeline with TP-Linker	0.3973	3.39%
Backbone with noisy entities	0.4018	3.8%
Backbone with KL loss	0.4047	4.13%
Backbone with relationship re-targeting	0.4044	4.1%
Backbone with all technical methods	0.4258	6.24%

4 Conclusions

In this paper, we propose a two-step pipeline consists of a TP-Liner and a PL-Marker to extract medical entities and relationships. The first step is to extract medical entities from medical texts, and the second step is to determine the relationships between these entities. Facing many challenges from medical inquiries mining task, we apply four technical methods to improve the performance of pipeline. Nevertheless, there still exists some potential methods to increase the robustness of the pipeline. Due to the truncation of fixed length, long-range entities could not be learned well. In addition, unlabeled data could help to train the models better when meeting dirty data.

References

1. Zihao, L., Mosha, C., Zhenxin, M., et al.: CMedCausal-Chinese medical causal relation extraction dataset. biomedrxiv. **43**(12), 23–27 (2022). https://doi.org/10.12201/bmr.202211.00004
2. Deming, Y., Yankai, L., Peng, L., et al.: Packed levitated marker for entity and relation extraction. In: Smaranda, M., Preslav, N., Aline, V. (eds.) Proceedings of the 60th Annual Meeting of the Association for Computational Linguistics (Volume 1: Long Papers), Dublin, May 2022, pp. 4904–4917 (2022)
3. Yucheng, W., Bowen, Y., Yueyang, Z., et al.: TPLinker: single-stage joint extraction of entities and relations through token pair linking. In: Donia, S., Nuria, B., Chengqing, Z. (eds.) Proceedings of the 28th International Conference on Computational Linguistics, Barcelona, December 2020, pp. 1572–1582 (2020)
4. Wenxuan, Z., Muhao, C.: Learning from noisy labels for entity-centric information extraction. In: Marie-Francine, M., Xuanjing, H., Lucia, S., et al. (eds.) Proceedings of the 2021 Conference on Empirical Methods in Natural Language Processing, Punta Cana, November 2021, pp. 5381–5392 (2021)
5. Jianlin, S.: GlobalPointer: A Unified Method for Nested and Non-nested Ner. https://kexue.fm/archives/8373 (2021). Accessed 10 Jan 2023
6. Jianlin, S.: GPLinker: GlobalPointer-based Joint Extraction of Entities. https://kexue.fm/archives/8888 (2022). Accessed 10 Jan 2023
7. Ahmed, F.G.: Evaluating Deep Learning Models: The Confusion Matrix, Accuracy, Precision, and Recall. https://blog.paperspace.com/deep-learning-metrics-precision-recall-accuracy (2021). Accessed 13 Jan 2023
8. Diederik, P.K., Jimmy, B.: Adam: A Method for Stochastic Optimization (2017). arXiv:1412.6980
9. Yinhan, L., Myle, O., Naman, G., et al.: RoBERTa: A Robustly Optimized BERT Pretraining Approach (2019). arXiv:1907.11692
10. Vikas, Y., Steven, B.: A survey on recent advances in named entity recognition from deep learning models. In: Emily, M.B., Leon, D., Pierre, I. (eds.) Proceedings of the 27th International Conference on Computational Linguistics, Santa Fe, August 2018, pp. 2145–2158 (2018)

A Multi-span-Based Conditional Information Extraction Model

Jiajia Jiang, Xiaowei Mao(✉), Ping Huang, Mingxing Huang, Xiaobo Zhou, Yao Hu, and Peng Shen

Beijing Waterdrop Technology Group Co., Ltd., Beijing, China
{jiangjiajia,maoxiaowei,huangping15,huangmingxing, zhouxiaobo,huyao,shenpeng}@shuidi-inc.com

Abstract. Conditional information extraction plays an important role in medical information extraction applications, such as medical information retrieval, medical knowledge graph construction, intelligent diagnosis and medical question-answering. Based on the evaluation task of China Conference on Health Information Processing 2022 (CHIP 2022), we propose a Multi-span-based Conditional Information Extraction model (MSCIE), which can well solve the conditional information extraction by extracting multiple span and the relations between each span. Moreover, the model provide a solution to conditional information extraction in complex scenes such as discontinuous entities, entity overlap, and entity nesting. Finally, our model, with the fusion of two pretrained models, has obtained the performance of the 1st in list A and the 2nd in list B, which also proves the effectiveness of the model.

Keywords: Causal Entity Information Extraction · Conditional Information Extraction

1 Introduction

In the field of information extraction [1], entity relations are typically represented as SPO (Subject, Predicate, Object) triples. However, in the medical field, a large amount of medical knowledge can only be satisfied under specific conditions (C), and the entity relation triplet cannot fully reflect the accuracy and reliability of knowledge. For example, the medication and treatment plans of the disease are related to the degree of the disease, and the symptoms are also related to the personal physical condition. Therefore, in the construction of medical knowledge graph, the extraction of conditions (C) has also become an indispensable part, the conditional information extraction task solution based on quadruple (S, P, O, C) has become the key to whether medical knowledge can be better and accurately applied.

The 8th China Health Information Processing Conference (CHIP 2022) [2] set up a medical causal entity relationship extraction task. In addition to the common causal relationship and hyponymy relationship in medical information

B. Tang et al. (Eds.): CHIP 2022, CCIS 1773, pp. 66–72, 2023.
https://doi.org/10.1007/978-981-99-4826-0_7

extraction, this task also adds conditional relationship extraction to modify specific causal relationships, so that knowledge expression is more accurate and more reliable in application. On the basis of this task, we propose the Multi-span-based Conditional Information Extraction model (MSCIE). By jointly extracting multiple span (used to represent entities) and the relationships between span (used to represent relationships between entities), we can obtain quadruple (S, P, O, C) to solve the conditional relationship extraction task. In addition, the model can also be extended to solve the conditional information extraction in complex scenes such as discontinuous entities and entity overlap, and has good usability. In CHIP2022 testing data, with the fusion of two pretrained models, our model has obtained the performance of the 1st in list A and the 2nd in list B in CHIP 2022, which also proves the effectiveness.

Next, the paper will introduce the data description, methodologies, experimental results and conclusions.

2 Data Description

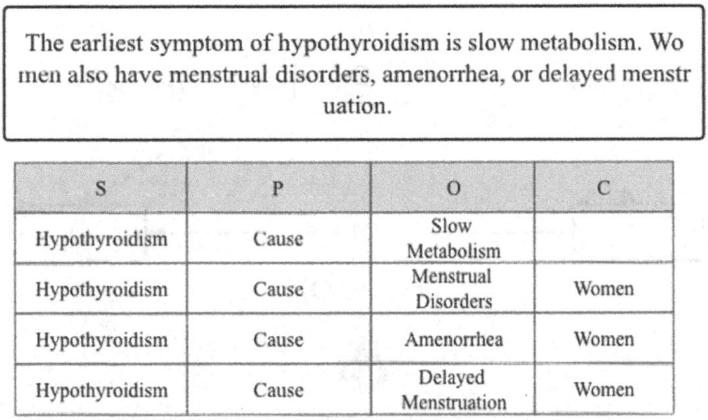

The earliest symptom of hypothyroidism is slow metabolism. Wo men also have menstrual disorders, amenorrhea, or delayed menstr uation.

S	P	O	C
Hypothyroidism	Cause	Slow Metabolism	
Hypothyroidism	Cause	Menstrual Disorders	Women
Hypothyroidism	Cause	Amenorrhea	Women
Hypothyroidism	Cause	Delayed Menstruation	Women

Fig. 1. An Example of Medical Causal Entity Relation

An example of medical causal entity relation is shown in Fig. 1. In this task[1] [10], a total of 1000 labeled data are provided for training, 1000 unlabeled data which can be used for helping model training, and 1000 test set A and B lists respectively. In the training set, the maximum length of the text is 544, the minimum length is 29, and the average length is 267.38. Among them, 7056 causal relations are unconditional, 659 causal relations are conditional, and 1089 are superior inferior relations.

[1] https://tianchi.aliyun.com/dataset/129573.

After data analysing, the following characteristics of this dataset need to be considered in the process of building our model and solution.

a) The length of the text is moderate and there is no too long data. The common length of the pretrained model is 512, which can meet the needs without special settings.
b) The data distribution is uneven, which should be considered.
c) The task is based on paragraph annotation, and there are crossing sentence relation annotations.
d) There are no discontinuous entities in annotations, and there are long annotations with multiple entities connected together.
e) In addition to the common triples (S, P, O), there are also quaternions (S, P, O, C) in the task.
f) The way to use the 1000 unlabeled data reasonably.

3 Methodologies

3.1 Model Architecture

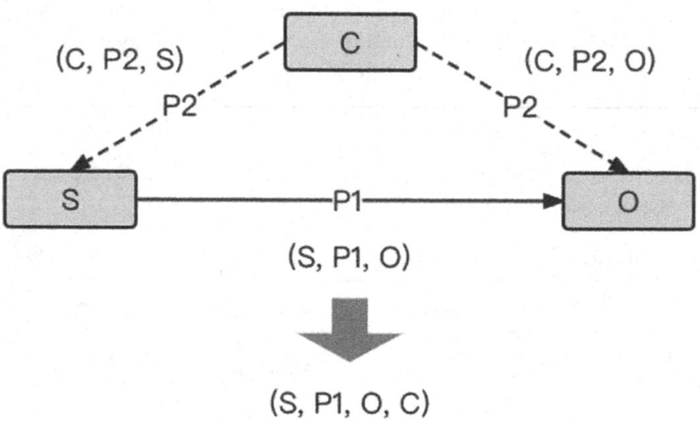

Fig. 2. An Example of a Quaternion

Firstly, the task can be represented by a quaternion (S, P, O, C), as shown in Fig. 2. It includes a common triplet (S, P1, O), as well as a conditional entity C and its conditional relations P2 with the head entity and tail entity. If there is a relation P1 between the head entity and the tail entity, a triple (S, P1, O) can be obtained. If an entity is related to the head entity and the tail entity of the triplet respectively, it can be considered that entity C is the conditional entity of the triplet (S, P1, O), so that we can get a quaternion (S, P1, O, C). Therefore, in this paper, the extraction of quaternions (S, P, O, C) is converted into the extraction task of multiple spans and the relations between each span. Each span is corresponded to an entity, and the relations between each span pair are corresponded to the relations between entities [13]. Based on above, we propose a multi-span-based conditional information extraction model in this paper.

For a text T with length L, the extraction task of this model can be divided into two parts, one is to extract entity spans, and the other is to extract the relations between spans.

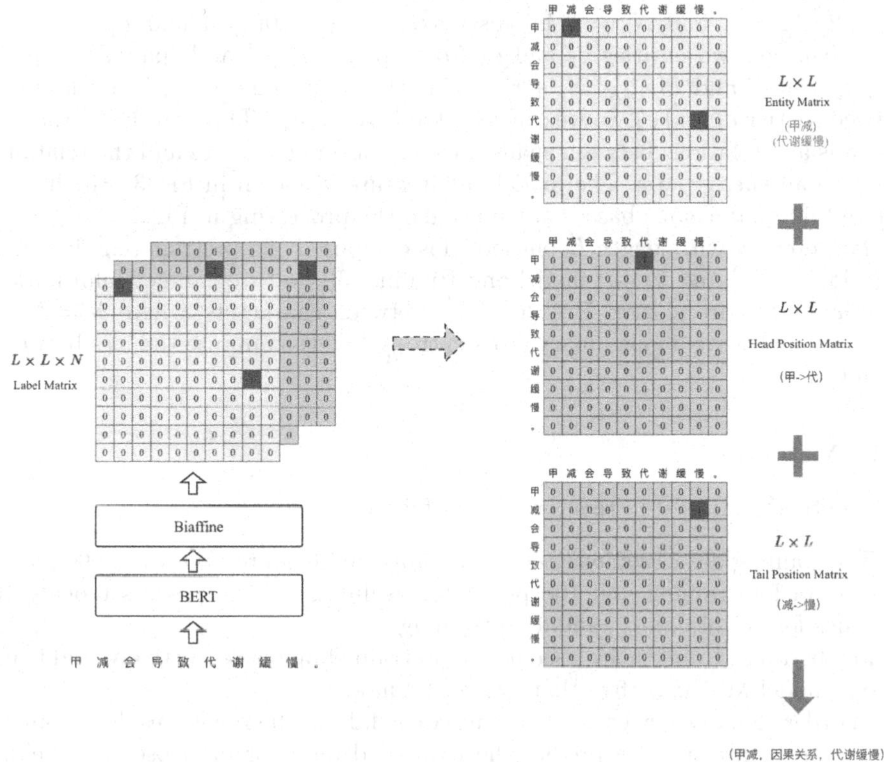

Fig. 3. Model Architecture

For the extraction of entity spans, the span based extraction method [3,11] is adopted. At first, we construct a span matrix $Re \in R^{L \times L \times N_e}$, where N_e is the number of entities. In this task $N_e = 1$, $Re \in R^{L \times L \times 1}$. if $Re[i, j, 0] = 1$, it means that the text span $T[i, j]$ with the starting position i and ending position j is an entity. Otherwise, the span $T[i, j]$ is not an entity.

For the extraction of entity relations, we adopt the same architecture and construct a relation matrix $Rr \in R^{L\times L\times(N_r\times 2)}$ [12], where N_r is the number of relations. In this task $N_r = 3$, $Rr \in R^{L\times L\times 6}$. For the relation r, if $Rr[i, j, r] = 1$, it means that there is a relation between the two spans, which one of them starts with the character $T[i]$ and the other starts with the character $T[j]$ respectively. if $Rr[i, j, N_r + r] = 1$, it means there is a relation between the two spans, which one of them ends with the character $T[i]$ and the other ends with the character $T[j]$ respectively. If the heads and tails of two spans have a same relation r, the two spans have a relation r. Other situations are similar.

Therefore, for the constructed label matrix $L \in R^{L\times L\times N}$, where $N = N_e + N_r \times 2$, $N_e = 1$ and $N_r = 3$ in this task, if $L[i_1, j_1, 0] = 1$ and $L[i_2, j_2, 0] = 1$, we can get two entities e_1 and e_2 from span $T[i_1, j_1]$ and span $T[i_2, j_2]$. If $L[i_1, i_2, r] = 1$ and $L[j_1, j_2, N_r + r] = 1$ at the same time, there is a relation r between entity e_1 and e_2. So we can get a triple (e_1, r, e_2). Through the extraction of spans and relations between spans, we can obtain all entities and the relations between all entity pairs. The model architecture is shown in Fig. 3. Finally, we can obtain quaternions based on triples like the processing in Fig. 2.

For a text T with length L, our model is composed of a pretrain (e.g. Roberta [4], Macbert [5] and so on) model and Biaffine [3], and we can get information interaction feature matrix $M \in R^{L\times L\times N}$ between characters, where $N = N_e + N_r \times 2$. Finally, we adopt binary cross entropy loss to compute the loss between L and M.

3.2 Method

The method proposed in this paper is as follows.

a) The training data 1000 pieces are randomly divided into two parts, 900 pieces of data for training and 100 pieces for evaluating. This process repeats 10 times for 10 fold cross validation training.
b) Macbert and Roberta are used as the pretrained model respectively, and train our model MSCIE. After that, we get 20 models.
c) In order to make better use of the unlabeled data, the model results obtained in step b) are used to predict the unlabeled data for data pseudo labeling [14]. Because the overall accuracy of the model is not high in this data set, only a small part of the data with high confidence is selected to add to the training set.
d) On the expanded training set in step c, Macbert and Roberta are also used as the pretrained model to train the model respectively. We also get 20 models.
e) We use the models obtained in steps b and d to predict the test set respectively, and vote for the final results to integrate different model prediction results. Finally, according to the precision and recall of the voting results, we adjust the voting threshold, and try to make the precision and recall rate close to each other, so as to obtain the optimal F1 value.

3.3 Model Expansion

In this task, it does not include relation extraction in complex scenes such as discontinuous entities, entity overlap, and entity nesting. However, in the actual medical scene, such complex relation extraction often exists. The multi-span-based conditional information extraction model proposed in this paper is also applicable to extracting relations in complex scenes.

For extraction of discontinuous entities, firstly we extract each span through the span matrix Re. After that, for the relation matrix Rr, we change the dimension of Rr to $L \times L \times \{(N_r + 1) \times 2\}$, where the added dimension is used to represent the discontinuous entity relation. If there is a discontinuous entity relation between span e_1 and e_2, the span e_1 and e_2 can compose a discontinuous entity. All discontinuous entities can be obtained in this way.

Because we adopt the binary cross entropy loss and build the labels with binary values, each span can have multiple relations with multiple spans. Base on this, our model can solve the relation extraction with entity overlap, and entity nesting.

4 Experiments

In experiments [10], to handle with data uneven distribution, improve model generalization and training speed, we adopt Focal Loss [6], Poly1 Focalloss [7], FGM [8], EMA [9], Automatic Mixed Precision training and so on. The final test results are as follows, ranking 1st in list A and 2nd in list B (Table 1).

Table 1. Experiment Results

Models	Dataset	List A	List B
Roberta-Large	train.json	0.4206	-
Macbert-Large	train.json	0.4077	-
Roberta-Large (10 fold)	train.json	0.4469	-
Macbert-Large (10 fold)	train.json	0.4272	-
Roberta-Large (10 fold) + Macbert-Large (10 fold)	train.json	0.4490	-
Roberta-Large (10 fold) + Macbert-Large (10 fold)	train*.json	0.4510	0.4355

* Add selected unlabeled data's predictions to the train data

5 Conclusion

In this paper, in order to make the extracted knowledge more accurate, reliable and highly available, we focus on conditional relation extraction in complex medical scenes and propose a multi-span-based conditional information extraction model (MSCIE). Through the joint extraction of multiple spans and the relations between spans, we can get the quaternions (S, P, O, C). We achieve good results in CHIP 2022, which proves the validity and practicability of the model proposed in this paper. For now, due to the limitation of data set, our model has not been verified in relation extraction under complex scenes such as discontinuous entities, entity overlap, and entity nesting, we only have made theoretical analysis. The future work will be to verify the model effect on more complex data.

References

1. Zong, H., Lei, J., Li, Z., et al.: Overview of technology evaluation dataset for medical multimodal information extraction. J. Med. Inform. **43**(12), 2–5+22 (2022)
2. Li, Z., Chen, M., Yin, K., et al.: CHIP 2022 shared task overview: medical causal entity relationship extraction. In: Health Information Processing: 8th China Conference, CHIP 2022, Hangzhou, China, October 21–23, 2022, Revised Selected Papers. Springer Nature Singapore, Singapore (2022)
3. Yu, J., Bohnet, B., Poesio, M.: Named entity recognition as dependency parsing. In: The 58th Annual Meeting of the Association for Computational Linguistics, pp. 6470–6476 (2020)
4. Cui, Y., et al.: Pre-training with whole word masking for Chinese BERT. arXiv preprint arXiv:1906.08101 (2019)
5. Cui, Y., et al.: Revisiting Pre-trained Models for Chinese Natural Language Processing. arXiv preprint arXiv:2004.13922 (2020)
6. Lin, T.-Y., Goyal, P., Girshick, R.B., He, K., Dollár, P.: Focal loss for dense object detection. IEEE Trans. Pattern Anal. Mach. Intell. **42**, 318–327 (2020)
7. Leng, Z., Tan, M., Liu, C., Cubuk, E.D., Shi, J., et al.: PolyLoss: a polynomial expansion perspective of classification loss functions. In: 10th International Conference on Learning Representations (2022)
8. Miyato, T., Dai, A.M., Goodfellow, I.: Adversarial training methods for semi-supervised text classification. arXiv preprint arXiv:1605.07725 (2016)
9. Goyal, P., Dollár, P., Girshick, R.,Noordhuis, P., et al.: Accurate, Large Minibatch SGD: Training ImageNet in 1 Hour. arXiv preprint arXiv:1706.02677v2 (2018)
10. Li, Z., Chen, M., Ma, Z., et al.: CMedCausal: Chinese medical causal relationship extraction dataset. J. Med. Inform. **43**(12), 23–27+31 (2022)
11. Li, J., Fei, H., Liu, J., et al.: Unified named entity recognition as word-word relation classification. In: Proceedings of the AAAI Conference on Artificial Intelligence, pp. 10965–10973 (2022)
12. Wang, Y., Yu, B., Zhang, Y., et al.: TPLinker: single-stage joint extraction of entities and relations through token pair linking. In: Proceedings of the 28th International Conference on Computational Linguistics, pp. 1572–1582 (2020)
13. Shang, Y.-M., Huang, H., Mao, X-L.: OneRel: joint entity and relation extraction with one module in one step. In: Proceedings of the AAAI Conference on Artificial Intelligence, pp. 11285–11293 (2022)
14. Rizve, M.N., Duarte, K., Rawat, Y.S., et al.: An uncertainty-aware pseudo-label selection framework for semi-supervised learning. In: International Conference on Learning Representations (2021)

Medical Causality Extraction: A Two-Stage Based Nested Relation Extraction Model

Yiwen Jiang[1(✉)] and Jingyi Zhao[2]

[1] Winning Health Technology Group Co., LTD., Shanghai, China
j_yw@winning.com.cn

[2] School of Economics and Management, Tongji University, Shanghai, China
2152165@tongji.edu.cn

Abstract. The extraction of medical causality contributes to constructing medical causal knowledge graphs, and enhancing the interpretability of modern medical consultation process. In this paper, we present our approach to medical causal entity and relation extraction in the 8th China Health Information Processing Conference (CHIP 2022) Open Shared Task. Nested relations and overlapping relations with shared entities are two major challenges in this task. We propose a two-stage model to achieve nested relation extraction. In the first stage, we extract traditional non-nested relations and explore how to utilize causal relational signals in entity recognition module to alleviate the problem of overlapping relations. In the second stage, we identify entities in nested relations through the method of machine reading comprehension and design a span-based contrastive learning method (SpanCL) with under-sampling strategy to determine whether causality is nested. The experiment results show that the method we proposed can achieve 43.23% in terms of macro-averaged F1-score.

Keywords: medical causality extraction · nested relation extraction · span-based contrastive learning

1 Introduction

Modern healthcare requires doctors to make patient-centered assessment, diagnosis and treatment with strong medical interpretability. Medical causality is logically a significant part of explainable medical consultation. To mine the knowledge of medical causality at scale from the source of text, a corpus named CMedCausal (Chinese Medical Causal dataset) [10] was developed as a benchmark dataset. As part of the 8th China Health Information Processing Conference (CHIP 2022) Open Shared Task[1] [11,23], the CMedCausal track[2] aims to extract cause-and-effect relationships for the subsequent construction of medical causal knowledge graphs or interpretation networks.

[1] http://www.cips-chip.org.cn/2022/eval2

[2] https://tianchi.aliyun.com/dataset/129573.

B. Tang et al. (Eds.): CHIP 2022, CCIS 1773, pp. 73–85, 2023.
https://doi.org/10.1007/978-981-99-4826-0_8

CMedCausal track is a Relation Extraction (RE) task in which three different relation types (i.e., causal, conditional and hyponymy relations) will be extracted among medical concept mentions. These medical concepts are clinical-finding-oriented (including inspection results) and disease-oriented entity spans. Three refined causality is defined as following: (1) Causal Relation: a cause directly leads to a result with no conditions mentioned. (2) Conditional Relation: a cause directly leads to a result under a certain condition. Note that the condition sets a premise for the causal relation as a whole, and the condition cannot directly induce the result without the cause. (3) Hyponymy Relation: an association between hypernyms and hyponyms, indicating different scopes of medical concepts. Normally, a hyponym is an instance of a hypernym, which is a broader concept of the hyponym. The CMedCausal Annotation Guideline [10] introduces that this task only focuses on first-order causality expressed explicitly in the text, ignoring those higher-order relations derived by causal inference.

Nested Relation Extraction (NRE) and Overlapping Relations (OR) are two characteristics also challenges of CMedCausal dataset. Typical RE tasks aims to extract relational triples in form of $(subject, relation, object)$ in which $subject$ and $object$ are two named entities. By contrast, according to the definition of relation type, the object of conditional relation is a causal relation instead of an entity, which makes the RE task of CMedCausal more complicated one. The conditional relation is a quintuple with a relation nested inside, which thus is called NRE task. In addition, there are many cases of OR in CMedCausal dataset, where different relations share the same entity. The semantic role of an entity mention might be both cause and effect, and it might also be a condition to describe other causalities. This character stems from the real scenario of medical interpretation process. For causal RE task, the character feature of an entity mention cannot logically determine its type in the triplets. Since contextual semantics are decisive features, how to utilize causality signals to identify entity types is a great starting point for the OR problem.

In this paper, we propose a two-stage model to achieve nested RE in CMedCausal dataset. Specifically, we regard the unconditional causality as a special case of conditional relation because both can be represented by a quintuple as (*condition*, *conditional relation*, *cause*, *causal relation*,*result*) in which *condition* is allowed to be an empty set. Based on this, our proposed two-stage model extracts causal relations and hyponymy relations in the first stage, and then, as a second step, identifies the condition entities for all these extracted causal relations. In stage one, we formulate joint entity and relation extraction as a type-specific table-filling problem. Similar to the idea of TPLinker [18], token-pair linking module is used to score each element in the table while handshaking tagging schema is referenced to decode relational triples. Moreover, we adopt Partition Filter Network (PFN) [20] to model balanced bi-directional interaction between Named Entity Recognition (NER) and RE tasks, so that causality signals can be used to identify entities to alleviate the OR problem. We formulate stage two as a

Machine Reading Comprehension (MRC) task. Each causal relation is regarded as a question of text, and the model is trained to answer the question through span extraction. Note that some questions are unanswerable due to no conditions. Besides, because of the observed imbalanced classification of conditional and unconditional causality in CMedCausal, we design an under-sampling strategy for a span-based contrastive learning method, enabling the model to learn conditional causality with relatively small sample size better. In summary, our contributions include:

1. We propose a two-stage model to solve NRE problem. Traditional RE method is used in stage one while MRC method in stage two. Besides, a span-based contrastive learning method with under-sampling strategy is designed to alleviate the problem of sample imbalance.
2. For OR problem, we use the encoder of PFN to bring causal signals into NER task module, and experimentally show the importance of relation signals.
3. We conduct experiments on CMedCausal test dataset, and the experimental results demonstrate the validity of our method. The macro-F1 score won the third place in CHIP 2022 CMedCausal track.

2 Related Work

The extraction of relational triples from unstructured natural language text is a fundamental task in information extraction and a crucial step in the construction of large-scale knowledge graphs such as Medical KG [9] and SMR KG [5] in the medical field.

At present, the mainstream approaches for relation extraction are based on joint extraction of entities and relations, which can be roughly classified into the following three categories. The first one is sequence labeling [8,19,22], which involves assigning one or more labels to each token in a sentence to locate the starting and ending positions of entities and relations. The second one is to enumerate all spans in a sentence and classify them (aka. table-filling based approach) [6,17,18]. This method creates a $L \times L$ table (L is the number of tokens in an input sentence) for each entity or relation type. Each element in the table represents an entity span or denotes the starting/ending positions of two entity pairs for specific relation type. In contrast to the previously discussed discriminative methods, there are some generative approaches based on Seq2Seq models [13,21]. These methods regard a triple as a token sequence and use an encoder-decoder architecture to generate multiple relational triples in a certain order. Although these methods can effectively extract entities and relations jointly, there is few research on nested relation extraction. In this work, we explore how to use table-filling based extraction method to solve nested relation extraction problem and propose a two-stage model for CMedCausal dataset.

3 Method

In this section, we describe our two-stage model designed for nested RE problem. The overall structure of the model is presented in Fig. 1. We begin by defining CMedCausal task. Then, we present the technical details of the method. Our proposed two-stage model architecture contains BERT Encoder [4] and Global Pointer Network (GPN) [15] at each stage. BERT is used to encode contextual representation of each token in input sequence. We adopt token-pair tagging method and utilize GPN as a basic token-pair linking unit for entity and relation prediction. Furthermore, in the first stage, the encoder of Partition Filter Network [20] is applied to ensure sufficient interaction and information sharing between NER and RE task units. For MRC model in the second stage, we propose a Span-based Contrastive Learning (SpanCL) method with under-sampling strategy to teach the model how to distinguish questions that can be answered from the ones that cannot.

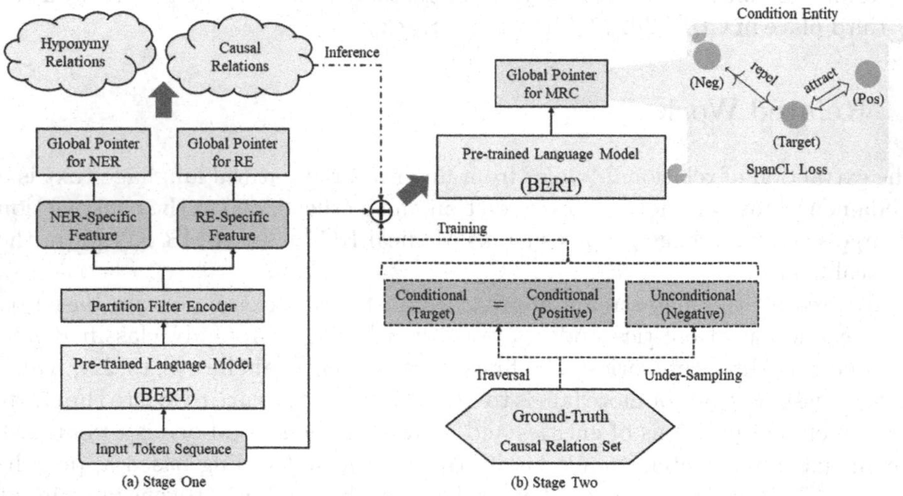

Fig. 1. The architecture and pipeline of the proposed two-stage model.

3.1 Problem Definition

Formally, given an input sentence $s = \{w_1, ..., w_L\}$ with L tokens, w_i denotes the i-th token of sequence s. CMedCausal task aims to extract three refined causalities i.e., causal, conditional and hyponymy relations. The non-nested hyponymy relation is denoted by (*hypernym*, *hyponymy relation*, *hyponym*), where *hypernym* and *hyponym* are two entities, represented in the form of token-pairs $\langle w_s, w_e \rangle$. The token-pair $\langle w_s, w_e \rangle$ signifies an entity span, starting with token w_s and ending with w_e. For nested conditional relation, it is denoted by (*condition*, *conditional relation*, *cause*, *causal relation*, *result*), where *condition*, *cause* and *result* are entities represented by the same token-pair method. When *condition* is an empty set, the conditional relation degenerates into an unconditional causal relation.

3.2 Token Pair Tagging Method

In stage one, we formulate joint entity and relation extraction as a type-specific table-filling problem. CMedCausal tasks are deconstructed into $1 + 2 \times |R|$ table-filling tasks, where $|R|$ denotes the number of relation types. Although the entities of CMedCausal have different semantic types e.g., cause, condition, etc., we do not distinguish them and fill out only one table whose element $e_{i,j}$ represents the score of a token-pair(w_i, w_j) is an entity span. For each relation, we create two tables, namely head-table and tail-table, corresponding to the scores of the first and the last token-pairs of the two entities respectively. The similar logic goes for element $r^l_{i,j}$ in relation-specific head/tail-table, where w_i and w_j represent the starting or ending token of subject and object entity with relation type l. Each table-filling task builds a $L \times L$ scoring matrix, where L is the length of input sentence. In this way, we can decode the relational triples $\langle w_x, w_y, l, w_m, w_n \rangle$ by querying multi-tables for token-pairs that satisfy following conditions:

$$e_{x,y} \geq \lambda_e; e_{m,n} \geq \lambda_e; r^l_{x,m} \geq \lambda_r; r^l_{y,n} \geq \lambda_r \tag{1}$$

where λ_e and λ_r are the threshold for prediction, both are set to 0 by default. Particularly, we only extract hyponymy and causal relations in the first stage, followed by the same tagging method to identify condition entities based on first-extracted causal relations in the second stage. We create one table for condition entity recognition and adopt the same token-pair linking unit in both stages.

3.3 BERT Encoder

The BERT model is a multi-layer bidirectional Transformer encoder [16] based on self-attention mechanism. BERT is pre-trained with two unsupervised tasks i.e., masked language model and next sentence prediction, on large-scale unannotated text datasets. The pre-trained model is then fine-turned to adapt to different downstream tasks, a process known as transfer learning. Given an input token sequence $s = w_1, w_2, ..., w_L$, after 12 stacked self-attention blocks, the output of BERT is a contextual representation sequence $H = h_1, h_2, ..., h_L$.

3.4 Global Pointer Network (GPN)

We adopt the architecture of GPN as the basic unit for token-pair linking module. Given a sentence encoding feature $H = h_1, ..., h_L$, for each token-pair (w_i, w_j), two feedforward layers are used to map head and tail token features h_i and h_j into low-dimensional vectors $q_{i,a}$ and $k_{j,a}$ as following:

$$\begin{aligned} q_{i,a} &= W_{q,a} h_i + b_{q,a} \\ k_{j,a} &= W_{k,a} h_j + b_{k,a} \end{aligned} \tag{2}$$

where $W_{q,a}$ and $W_{k,a}$ are parameter matrixes, as well as $b_{q,a}$ and $b_{k,a}$ are bias vectors for specific type α to be learned during training. Then, the score of the token-pair that leverages the relative positions through a multiplicative attention mechanism, is calculated by Eq. (3).

$$S_\alpha(i,j) = (R_i q_{i,a})^T (R_j k_{j,a}) \tag{3}$$

Rotary position embedding [14] is applied into the score calculation, which satisfies $R_i^T R_j = R_{j-1}$.

3.5 Partition Filter Encoder (PFE) in Stage One

The encoder of Partition Filter Network is a recurrent feature encoder and is inserted between the BERT encoder and the GPN module in order to generate task-specific features based on shared input sequence H. At each time step, this module follows two sub-steps: partition and filter. PFE first partitions each neuron into task-specific partitions and inter-task shared partition, according to its contribution to individual tasks, and then different partitions are combined to filter task-irrelevant information.

Partition. For each time step t, similar to LSTM, a hidden state and a cell state with history information are denoted by h_t and c_t. In addition, given input token x_t, a candidate cell $\widetilde{c_t}$ is calculated through linear transformation and activation function:

$$\widetilde{c_t} = tanh(Linear([x_t; h_{t-1}])) \tag{4}$$

Entity gate $\widetilde{e}$ and relation gate $\widetilde{r}$ are leveraged for neuron partition. The gates are calculated using cummax activation function $cummax(\cdot) = cumsum(softmax(\cdot))$ as following:

$$\begin{aligned} \widetilde{e} &= cummax(Linear([x_t; h_{t-1}])) \\ \widetilde{r} &= 1 - cummax(Linear([x_t; h_{t-1}])) \end{aligned} \tag{5}$$

Two gates naturally divide neurons for current candidate cell state $\widetilde{c_t}$ and historical cell state c_{t-1}, respectively into three partitions in the same manner. The calculation for c_{t-1} is shown in Eq. (6). Three partitions include two task partitions, namely entity partition $\rho_{e,c_{t-1}}$ and relation partition $\rho_{r,c_{t-1}}$, storing intra-task information, as well as one shared partition $\rho_{s,c_{t-1}}$ to store inter-task information that is valuable to both NER and RE tasks.

$$\begin{aligned} \rho_{s,c_{t-1}} &= \widetilde{e}_{c_{t-1}} \circ \widetilde{r}_{c_{t-1}} \\ \rho_{e,c_{t-1}} &= \widetilde{e}_{c_{t-1}} - \rho_{s,c_{t-1}} \\ \rho_{r,c_{t-1}} &= \widetilde{r}_{c_{t-1}} - \rho_{s,c_{t-1}} \end{aligned} \tag{6}$$

Finally, each type of partition from both target cells are aggregated to form three partitioned results: ρ_e, ρ_r and ρ_s through Eq. (7).

$$\rho = \rho_{c_{t-1}} \circ c_{t-1} + \rho_{\widetilde{c}_t} \circ \widetilde{c}_t \tag{7}$$

Filter. Information in entity partition and shared partition are combined to form entity memory denoted by μ_e, where $\mu_e = \rho_e + \rho_s$. Information in relation partition ρ_r is assumed to be irrelevant or even harmful to NER task and thus, is filtered out. The same logic applies to relation memory $\mu_r = \rho_r + \rho_s$. The shared memory is evenly accessible to both entity memory and relation memory, ensuring balanced interaction between different tasks. At last, three memories are used to form cell state c_t and hidden state h_t, which will be the input to next time step.

$$\begin{aligned} c_t &= LayerNorm(Linear([\mu_{e,t}; \mu_{r,t}; \mu_{s,t}])) \\ h_t &= tanh(c_t) \end{aligned} \tag{8}$$

In Eq. (8), layer normalization is applied to prevent gradient explosion and stabilize the training process. These two memory blocks μ_e and μ_r are further activated and combined with corresponding global representation to form task-specific features h_e and h_r for NER and RE tasks respectively, which are subsequently fed to the corresponding GPN modules.

3.6 MRC Model in Stage Two

The second stage is an MRC task. Each causal relation is regarded as a question of the text, and each span is scored by the same token-pair linking module, GPN, as the first stage. Given a relational triple $\langle w_x, w_y, l, w_m, w_n \rangle$, where $a_1 = \{w_x, ..., w_y\}$ is a subject (cause) entity, $a_2 = \{w_m, ..., w_n\}$ is an object (result) entity, and $l = causal\ relation$. We concatenate the given s, a_1 and a_2 with classification token $[CLS]$ and separator token $[SEP]$ in BERT as the input sequence: $[CLS]\ s\ [SEP]\ a_1\ [SEP]\ a_2\ [SEP]$. In addition, to help the model locate the start position of a_1 and a_2 mentioned in s, we change the position encoding of a_1 and a_2 to be exactly the same as those mentions in the original text. The output of the BERT model is then fed to the GPN to score each span. The entity span with achieving the highest score and exceeding a pre-defined threshold $\lambda_e = 0$ is selected as the answer. If none of the spans satisfies the aforementioned requirements, then the question is unanswerable, implying an unconditional causal relation.

Span-Based Contrastive Learning (SpanCL) Method. The aim of SpanCL method with under-sampling strategy is to improve model's capability of distinguish unanswerable questions and alleviate the problem of sample imbalance. Given an input sentence s, we treat each ground-truth conditional causal relation $\langle a_1, a_2 \rangle \in C$ as an anchor. We first introduce how the positive and negative examples are generated.

- **Positive examples.** Inspired by the idea of R-Drop [12], we feed the same input to the model twice, due to the dropout layers that randomly drop neurons, different sub-models will generate two different distributions, one of which we consider to be the positive example of the anchor.
- **Negative examples.** We randomly sample a causal relation $\langle b_1, b_2 \rangle \in U$, where U represents the ground-truth collection of unconditional causal relations. Next, $\langle b_1, b_2 \rangle$ is concatenated with sentence s to form the negative example. For most input texts in the CMedCausal dataset, $|U| \gg |C|$, and thus an under-sampling strategy. In case $U = \emptyset$, then two random spans will be sampled from s to form a negative example.

We improve MRC models by contrasting causal relations according to their span representations of condition entities. Each span $\{w_i, ...w_j\}$ is reduced to a token-pair (w_i, w_j) in the scoring process of GPN, where the concatenation of vectors q_i and k_j is regarded as the span representation denoted by $z_{(i,j)} = [q_i; k_j]$. During training, given an answer condition entity (w_s, w_e) as an anchor for the question causal relation Q_{ach}, we generate a positive example Q_{pos} and a negative example Q_{neg} through the method introduced previously. Then (w_s, w_e) is the answer span to both Q_{ach} and Q_{pos} but not to Q_{neg}. The SpanCL loss is calculated as:

$$SpanCL\ loss = -log \frac{exp\left(\frac{\varphi\left(z_{(s,e)}^{Q_{ach}}, z_{(s,e)}^{Q_{pos}}\right)}{\tau}\right)}{exp\left(\frac{\varphi\left(z_{(s,e)}^{Q_{ach}}, z_{(s,e)}^{Q_{pos}}\right)}{\tau}\right) + exp\left(\frac{\varphi\left(z_{(s,e)}^{Q_{ach}}, z_{(s,e)}^{Q_{neg}}\right)}{\tau}\right)} \tag{9}$$

where $\varphi(u, v) = u^T v / \|u\| \cdot \|v\|$ is the cosine similarity between vectors u and v, $\tau > 0$ is a scalar temperature parameter.

3.7 Training Details and Inference

Since the matrix of each typed table in both stages is extremely sparse, we use Class Imbalance Loss [15] during training. The total loss is calculated as the sum of losses from all task tables:

$$log\left(1 + \sum_{(i,j)\in\Omega_{neg}^{a}} e^{-s_a\ (i,j)}\right) + log\left(1 + \sum_{(i,j)\in\Omega_{pos}^{a}} e^{s_a\ (i,j)}\right) \tag{10}$$

where (i, j) represent a token-pair (w_i, w_j), Ω_{neg}^a represents a collection of token-pairs that do not belong to type a, Ω_{pos}^a represents a collection of token-pairs whose entity type or relation type is a. In particular, formula (10) is a simplified version, when the threshold λ_e and λ_r are both 0. Moreover, in stage two, we traverse all ground-truth conditional causal relations for training and the final objective loss of MRC model is the sum of class imbalance loss and SpanCL loss. During inference, we use the causal relations extracted in the first stage.

4 Experiment

In this section, we provide data distribution details of CMedCausal dataset, the leaderboard performance and an analysis of the effect of proposed method.

4.1 CMedCausal Dataset

The CMedCausal dataset consists of 4,000 medical text data, with 2,000 used for model training and 2,000 for testing. The training corpus contains 1,000 labeled data and 1,000 unlabeled data, where the unlabeled data is allowed to be manually annotated or labeled using the pseudo-label method. The test dataset includes 1,000 data, which are used for final evaluation.

Table 1. Statistics for entity and relation types in the CMedCausal training set.

# of Roles for an Entity	Training Set
single	10,236
multiple (≥2)	1,257
# of Relation Types	**Training Set**
causal relation	7,056
conditional relation	659
hyponymy relation	1,089

Table 1 illustrates the distribution of entities and relations in the CMedCausal training set. It shows that 89% of entities have a single semantic role in context, while the remaining 11% have multiple roles, e.g., potentially both as cause and effect, since they are shared entities in overlapping relations. The relation distribution is imbalanced over the relation types, e.g., 8.5% of causalities are conditional, that is nested.

4.2 Experimental Setup

We randomly split the labeled dataset into train and development datasets with the ratio of 4:1. The training set is utilized to learn model parameters, while the development set is utilized to select optimal hyperparameters. We first applied the models trained on 1,000 labeled data to infer labels for the remaining 1,000 unlabeled data in the training set, creating pseudo-labels. These pseudo-labels are then merged with the original labeled data to form a new training corpus. The CMedCausal track is evaluated by the macro-averaged F1-score of three relation types. We employed a five-fold cross-validation approach to apply ensemble learning to multiple models and evaluated the final performance of our proposed two-stage models on the test set.

4.3 Implementation and Hyperparameters

We tried different variants of the large-level BERT model, including RoBERTa [2], MacBERT [1] and PERT [3]. For all of these pre-trained models, we employed the same set of following hyperparameters without any further fine-tuning. Each training sample is pruned to at most 512 tokens. For both stages, we used a batch size of 24 and employed the hierarchical learning rate in the training process with Adam optimizer [7], using a learning rate of $1e-5$ for pre-trained weights and $1e-4$ for other weights. We trained for at most 100 epochs with early stopping strategy based on the performance of development set. Training stops when the F1-score on the development set fails to improve for 10 consecutive epochs or the maximum number of epochs has been reached. To prevent overfitting and generate positive examples, dropout layers with a dropout rate of 0.1 are used. The dimensions of the hidden vectors for PFE and GPN are set to 512 and 128 respectively. In the first stage, we combined the predictions of 15 models, which are trained using five-fold cross-validation on three pre-trained models. In the second stage, we only used 5 models trained by RoBERTa for ensemble.

Table 2. Model results in development set with different pre-trained models.

Model	Macro-F1 (Stage One)	F1 (Stage Two)
RoBERTa$_{large}$	61.99	32.65
MacBERT$_{large}$	61.34	28.86
PERT$_{large}$	60.29	28.40

4.4 Results

Table 2 presents the results of the two stages of different pre-trained models, with the average scores obtained in development set through five-fold cross-validation. The large-level RoBERTa model yields the highest performance, achieving F1 scores of 61.99% and 32.65% in the two stages. It is worth noting that MacBERT and PERT, while included in the experimental results for stage two, are not ultimately included in the final ensemble process.

Table 3. Precision (P), Recall (R) and F1 scores in test set of CMedCausal.

Relation Name	P	R	F1
causal relation	64.21	54.25	58.81
conditional relation	9.58	16.27	12.06
hyponymy relation	63.98	54.41	58.80
Overall	45.92	41.64	43.23

The results for final evaluation are summarized in Table 3. The causal relations, i.e., questions, used for MRC inference during the second stage are inferred by multiple models trained in the first stage and combined in an ensemble. In the development set, the F1-score of the conditional entity predicted based on the ground-truth causal labels can reach 32.65%. However, a significant discrepancy is observed in the test set, with an F1-score of only 12.06%, indicating that our proposed two-stage method experiences significant error propagation. Our proposed model ended up in third place on the leaderboard with a final overall macro-F1 score of 43.23%.

4.5 Ablation Study

To evaluate the validity of each component of our approach, we conducted ablation experiments using base-level RoBERTa on the development set. As illustrated in Table 4, incorporating PFE in the first stage can effectively enhance model's performance, demonstrating that information sharing between NER and RE tasks can alleviate the OR problem. Additionally, in the tagging and decoding processes for relational triples, we use both head and tail tables. Our comparison of methods that utilize either head or tail tables exclusively for decoding shows that using both head and tail tables can more accurately identify entity boundaries. For stage two, SpanCL is effective for the model's performance, and it increases the F1 score by 4.51%.

Table 4. Ablation study in development set.

Stage One	**Macro-F1**
RoBERTa_{base}	58.93
w/o PFE	56.56
w/ Head Only	58.02
w/ Tail Only	58.27
Stage Two	**F1**
RoBERTa_{base}	26.46
w/o SpanCL	21.95

5 Conclusion and Discussion

In this paper, we proposed a two-stage nested relation extraction method for extracting medical causalities from texts. In the first stage, we used the GPN for joint entity and relation extraction of non-nested causal and hyponymy relations. The second stage involves identifying the condition entities of causal relations through MRC method to achieve nested relation extraction. Our experiments demonstrated that PFE can effectively model the interactions between entities and relations, alleviating the issue of overlapping relations with shared entities. Additionally, we found that SpanCL, a training method based on under-sampling strategy, can improve the model's ability to distinguish between answered and unanswered questions, mitigating the class imbalance problem. However, our method inevitably suffers from error propagation. In the future, it will be worth researching how to develop a unified end-to-end model for extracting nested relations.

References

1. Cui, Y., Che, W., Liu, T., Qin, B., Wang, S., Hu, G.: Revisiting pre-trained models for Chinese natural language processing. In: Proceedings of the 2020 Conference on Empirical Methods in Natural Language Processing: Findings, pp. 657–668. Association for Computational Linguistics, Online, November 2020
2. Cui, Y., Che, W., Liu, T., Qin, B., Yang, Z.: Pre-training with whole word masking for Chinese BERT. IEEE/ACM Trans. Audio Speech Lang. Process. **29**, 3504–3514 (2021)
3. Cui, Y., Yang, Z., Liu, T.: Pert: pre-training BERT with permuted language model. arXiv preprint arXiv:2203.06906 (2022)
4. Devlin, J., Chang, M.W., Lee, K., Toutanova, K.: BERT: pre-training of deep bidirectional transformers for language understanding. In: Proceedings of the 2019 Conference of the North American Chapter of the Association for Computational Linguistics: Human Language Technologies, Volume 1 (Long and Short Papers), pp. 4171–4186. Association for Computational Linguistics, Minneapolis, Minnesota, June 2019
5. Gong, F., Wang, M., Wang, H., Wang, S., Liu, M.: SMR: medical knowledge graph embedding for safe medicine recommendation. Big Data Res. **23**, 100174 (2021)
6. Gupta, P., Schütze, H., Andrassy, B.: Table filling multi-task recurrent neural network for joint entity and relation extraction. In: Proceedings of COLING 2016, the 26th International Conference on Computational Linguistics: Technical Papers, pp. 2537–2547. The COLING 2016 Organizing Committee, Osaka, Japan, December 2016
7. Kingma, D., Ba, J.: Adam: A method for stochastic optimization. In: International Conference on Learning Representations, December 2014
8. Lample, G., Ballesteros, M., Subramanian, S., Kawakami, K., Dyer, C.: Neural architectures for named entity recognition. In: Proceedings of the 2016 Conference of the North American Chapter of the Association for Computational Linguistics: Human Language Technologies, pp. 260–270. Association for Computational Linguistics, San Diego, California, June 2016
9. Li, L., et al.: Real-world data medical knowledge graph: construction and applications. Artif. Intell. Med. **103**, 101817 (2020)
10. Li, Z., et al.: CMedCausal: Chinese medical causal relationship extraction dataset. J. Med. Inform. **43**(12), 23–27 (2022)
11. Li, Z., Chen, M., Yin, K.: CHIP 2022 shared task overview: medical causal entity relationship extraction. In: Health Information Processing: 8th China Conference. CHIP 2022, pp. 21–23. Springer Nature Singapore, Hangzhou, China, October 2022
12. Liang, X., et al.: R-drop: regularized dropout for neural networks. In: Advances in Neural Information Processing Systems, vol. 34, pp. 10890–10905. Curran Associates, Inc. (2021)

13. Lu, Y., et al.: Unified structure generation for universal information extraction. In: Proceedings of the 60th Annual Meeting of the Association for Computational Linguistics (Volume 1: Long Papers), pp. 5755–5772. Association for Computational Linguistics, Dublin, Ireland, May 2022
14. Su, J., Lu, Y., Pan, S., Wen, B., Liu, Y.: Roformer: enhanced transformer with rotary position embedding. arXiv preprint arXiv:2104.09864 (2021)
15. Su, J., et al.: Global pointer: novel efficient span-based approach for named entity recognition. arXiv preprint arXiv:2208.03054 (2022)
16. Vaswani, A., et al.: Attention is all you need. In: Advances in Neural Information Processing Systems. vol. 30. Curran Associates, Inc. (2017)
17. Wadden, D., Wennberg, U., Luan, Y., Hajishirzi, H.: Entity, relation, and event extraction with contextualized span representations. In: Proceedings of the 2019 Conference on Empirical Methods in Natural Language Processing and the 9th International Joint Conference on Natural Language Processing (EMNLP-IJCNLP), pp. 5784–5789. Association for Computational Linguistics, Hong Kong, China, November 2019
18. Wang, Y., Yu, B., Zhang, Y., Liu, T., Zhu, H., Sun, L.: TPLinker: single-stage joint extraction of entities and relations through token pair linking. In: Proceedings of the 28th International Conference on Computational Linguistics, pp. 1572–1582. International Committee on Computational Linguistics, Barcelona, Spain (Online), December 2020
19. Wei, Z., Su, J., Wang, Y., Tian, Y., Chang, Y.: A novel cascade binary tagging framework for relational triple extraction. In: Proceedings of the 58th Annual Meeting of the Association for Computational Linguistics, pp. 1476–1488. Association for Computational Linguistics, Online, July 2020
20. Yan, Z., Zhang, C., Fu, J., Zhang, Q., Wei, Z.: A partition filter network for joint entity and relation extraction. In: Proceedings of the 2021 Conference on Empirical Methods in Natural Language Processing, pp. 185–197. Association for Computational Linguistics, Online and Punta Cana, Dominican Republic, November 2021
21. Zeng, X., Zeng, D., He, S., Liu, K., Zhao, J.: Extracting relational facts by an end-to-end neural model with copy mechanism. In: Proceedings of the 56th Annual Meeting of the Association for Computational Linguistics (Volume 1: Long Papers), pp. 506–514. Association for Computational Linguistics, Melbourne, Australia, July 2018
22. Zheng, S., Wang, F., Bao, H., Hao, Y., Zhou, P., Xu, B.: Joint extraction of entities and relations based on a novel tagging scheme. In: Proceedings of the 55th Annual Meeting of the Association for Computational Linguistics (Volume 1: Long Papers), pp. 1227–1236. Association for Computational Linguistics, Vancouver, Canada, July 2017
23. Zong, H., et al.: Overview of technology evaluation dataset for medical multimodal information extraction. J. Med. Inform. **43**(12), 2–5 (2022)

Medical Decision Tree Extraction from Unstructured Text

Extracting Decision Trees from Medical Texts: An Overview of the Text2DT Track in CHIP2022

Wei Zhu[1], Wenfeng Li[1], Xiaoling Wang[1](✉), Wendi Ji[1], Yuanbin Wu[1], Jin Chen[2], Liang Chen[3], and Buzhou Tang[4]

[1] East China Normal University, Shanghai, China
xlwang@cs.ecnu.edu.cn
[2] University of Kentucky Lexington, Lexington, KY, USA
[3] Huashan Hospital of Fudan University, Shanghai, China
[4] Harbin Institute of Technology Shenzhen, Shenzhen, China

Abstract. This paper presents an overview of the Text2DT shared task[1] held in the CHIP-2022 shared tasks. The shared task addresses the challenging topic of automatically extracting the medical decision trees from the un-structured medical texts such as medical guidelines and textbooks. Many teams from both industry and academia participated in the shared tasks, and the top teams achieved amazing test results. This paper describes the tasks, the datasets, evaluation metrics, and the top systems for both tasks. Finally, the paper summarizes the techniques and results of the evaluation of the various approaches explored by the participating teams.[1](http://cips-chip.org.cn/2022/eval3)

Keywords: Text2DT · Information extraction · Pretrained models

1 Introduction

The novel task of extracting medical decision trees from medical texts (Text2DT) is proposed in [2]. Text2DT is defined as an automated task to explore the automatic extraction of MDTs from medical texts such as medical guidelines and textbooks. As illustrated in Fig. 1, the objective of this task is: given a real Chinese medical text, the model needs to return a MDT that models the medical rules in the text. To help to develop models that can complete this task, Text2DT [2] structures and normalizes a specific tree structure to model medical decision knowledge and constructs the first Text-to-MDT dataset in Chinese with 500 data pairs with the participation of medical experts and well-trained annotators.

The Text2DT task is essential for the development of Clinical decision support systems (CDSSs), the computer systems that use medical decision rules and knowledge to enhance healthcare-related decisions and behaviors [15,19,23]. The core of building a CDSS is the knowledge of the medical decision process, which are rules that link given conditions to medical decisions [8] and are

B. Tang et al. (Eds.): CHIP 2022, CCIS 1773, pp. 89–102, 2023.
https://doi.org/10.1007/978-981-99-4826-0_9

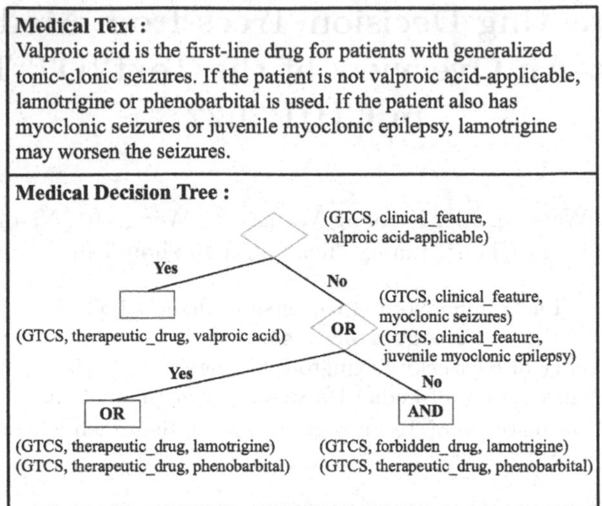

Fig. 1. An example of a MDT contained in a medical text from an epilepsy clinical guideline. "GTCS" is the abbreviation of "patient with generalized tonic-clonic seizures".

usually modeled as medical decision trees (MDTs). However, existing methods for constructing MDTs rely on manual tree construction by medical experts [18], which is time-consuming, laborious, and cannot absorb the latest research timely. All these hinder the construction, dissemination, maintenance of large-scale CDSSs [17]. Thus, the development of Text2DT systems can greatly facilitate the advancements of CDSSs.

However, as a novel complex information extraction task, Text2DT presents challenges for the current state-of-the-art models due the following reasons: 1) the current MDT lacks a normalized and structured form, leading to ambiguity in understanding medical decision knowledge and therefore hinders automated knowledge extraction; 2) the NLP community lacks benchmark data for training and validating MDT extraction tasks; and constructing such data is challenging in that annotating medical decision trees requires in-depth domain knowledge.

To facilitate the research into the Text2DT task, we have hosted the shared task of Text2DT as the 3rd shared task of the 8th China Conference on Health Information Processing (CHIP2022) [1]. By hosting this shared task, we are able to elicit strong or promising solutions to our novel shared task. The rest of papers are organized as follows. First, we will introduce our dataset, including the construction, data statistics, evaluation metrics. Then, we present the participation statistics and the official test results for the shared tasks. Finally, we analyze the top performing systems and their methodologies and form our findings.

2 Related Work

2.1 Medical Knowledge Extraction

Datasets on the extraction of medical entities and their relations in a given medical text have been released [24,29] for knowledge base construction or the needs of intelligent medicine. However, the limitations in the expressiveness of triplets prevent them from modeling more complex knowledge (e.g., the knowledge of the medical decision process). To model more complex knowledge, [11] introduced the role of "condition" and argued that a fact triplet is established based on some conditional triplets in the biomedical field. They focused on extracting fact triplets and their corresponding condition triplets in the text and recruited domain experts to annotate the dataset. However, this work only extracts all fact triplets and condition triplets in a sentence. Still, it cannot obtain the correspondence between them and cannot handle the complex situation in which the decision is made after multiple conditional judgments in medical decision-making.

2.2 Text2Tree Task

Many NLP tasks aim to extract trees from texts that can express their deep semantics, such as syntax trees, mathematical expressions, SQL statements [16,25,28]. Compared with other trees, MDTs are mainly different in the following three aspects: 1) Different application scenarios. MDTs are mainly oriented toward the medical decision process. It is necessary or helpful to consider medical knowledge for constructing the dataset and the model's design compared to other work. 2) Different granularity of nodes. The nodes of other trees are often a token, a number, or a symbol, and individual nodes have no specific meaning. Each node in the MDT is composed of triplets and the logical relationship between them, which already contains medical knowledge and clinical significance. 3) Different meanings of the tree structure. According to different judgment results, the decision tree will move from the root node to a leaf node. This leaf node represents the final decision and is also the final goal of the decision-making process. In contrast, other trees are continuously aggregated upward by leaf nodes and finally aggregated to the root node for the deep semantic expression of the text.

3 Evaluation Task Definition

3.1 Text2DT Task

As shown in Fig. 1, Text2DT focuses on the automatic extraction of MDTs from unstructured texts, as defined as follows:

Definition 1. ***(Text2DT):*** *Text2DT is a task, which aims at extracting a MDT from a given clinical medical text, where clinical medical texts are texts from clinical guidelines or medical textbooks that contain medical decision rules, and MDTs model the medical decision rules in the texts.*

Specifically, we denote a clinical medical text with n_text words as $X = [x_1, x_2, ..., x_{n\_text}]$, the goal of Text2DT is to generate the pre-order sequence of the nodes in the MDT $T = [N_1, N_2, ..., N_{n\_node}]$. The pre-order sequence of the nodes in the MDT can uniquely represent this tree, which is explained in detail in Sect. 3.2.

3.2 Medical Decision Tree

Condition Node and Decision Node. Nodes in a MDT consist of three parts: role, triplets, and logical relationship between triplets. We denote a node by

$$N = \{\Diamond/\Box,\ l(t_1, t_2, ..., t_{n\_tri})\}$$

where $\Diamond$ ($\Box$) denotes the node is a condition (decision) node, i.e., the node represents making a condition judgment (medical decision); $t = (subject, relation, object)$ is a triplet used to describe clinical knowledge or information; $l \in (and, or, null)$ denotes the logical relationship from t_1 to t_{n_tri} (note that $l = null$ if and only if the number of triplets is 1, i.e., $n = 1$); and $l(f_1, f_2, ..., f_n)$ denotes the content for making medical decisions or making condition judgments.

Tree Structure. A medical decision tree represents a simplified decision-making process meaning that the next condition judgment or decision is made according to the different results of the current condition judgment. Once a decision is made, the medical process is terminated. Therefore, we define a MDT as a binary tree consisting of condition and decision nodes, where non-leaf nodes are called conditional nodes, and leaf nodes are decision nodes. For the condition node, when the conditional judgment result is "Yes" ("No"), it will go to the left (right) branch for the next condition judgment or decision. It should be noted that each condition node has left and right child nodes. If the subsequent operation that needs to be done after the result of the condition judgment is "Yes" ("No") is not reflected in the text, a decision node without triplets is used as the left (right) child node. After this operation, a decision tree can be represented by a preorder sequence of its nodes.

Figure 1 shows an example of MDT. In the example, the medical decision process embedded in the medical text above can be modeled by the MDT below: 1) Firstly, the condition "whether valproic acid is applicable for patients with generalized tonic-clonic seizures" is determined, and if the result is "Yes," i.e., valproic acid is applicable, then go to the left branch and make the corresponding decision, i.e., valproic acid is used for treatment; 2) if the result is "No," that is, valproic acid is not applicable, next go to the right branch and make another conditional judgment, i.e., the condition "whether the patient has myoclonic seizures or suspected juvenile myoclonic epilepsy" is determined, and go to different branches according to the result.

3.3 Evaluation Metrics

The accuracy of MDT extraction **(Tree_Acc)** is used as our most stringent evaluation metric, a MDT is correct when it is precisely the same as the ground truth. Tree_Acc is calculated as follows:

$$\text{Tree\_Acc} = \frac{C}{N}$$

where C is the number of MDTs correctly extracted by the model and N is the total number of MDTs.

Since this overly strict metric affects the fairness of the evaluation, we propose four evaluation metrics from different perspectives:

1) **Triplet_F1**: Since the semantics of conditions and decisions are primarily expressed by triplets, we use the F1 score of triplet extraction as one of evaluation metrics.
2) **Node_F1**: Nodes are the main components of the MDT, so the F1 score of node extraction is used as one of evaluation metrics.
3) **DP_F1**: we call the path of a tree from the root node to a leaf node a decision path. A decision tree contains multiple decision paths. Since a complete decision path is meaningful for clinical decision-making, we use the F1 score of decision paths as an evaluation metric. The above three metrics are calculated as follows:

$$F1 = 2 \cdot \frac{precision \cdot recall}{precision + recall}$$

where *precision* is the proportion of correct triplets/nodes/decision paths extracted by the model to the total number of triplets/nodes/decision paths extracted by the model, *recall* is the proportion of correct triplets/nodes/decision extracted by the model to the total number of triplets/nodes/decision paths in the ground truth.
4) **Edit_DT**: similar to the edit distance of a string, the edit distance in the MDT is the minimum number of tree editing operations required to convert from one tree to another. The tree editing operation includes: inserting and deleting nodes, inserting and deleting triplets, and modifying the logical relationships between triplets. The edit distance of decision trees reflects the similarity between the extracted tree and the ground truth. Edit_DT is calculated as follows:

$$Edit\_DT = \frac{\sum_{i=1}^{n} Edit_i}{N}$$

where $Edit_i$ is the edit distance of the i-th MDT extracted by the model.

4 Evaluation Dataset

4.1 Data Collection

The Text2DT dataset was derived from clinical medicine textbooks and clinical practice guidelines. Clinical medicine textbooks are written by medical professionals under the guidance of the Ministry of Health and are extremely authoritative and reliable. Clinical practice guidelines are systematic medical guidelines to help doctors and patients choose the appropriate treatment based on specific clinical situations, and are structured, informative and up-to-date.

For the source data, we used both section-based and trigger/template-based filtering to locate segments containing knowledge of the medical decision process. Firstly, we selected chapters such as 'Treatment', 'Drug selection' and 'Medical solutions' in the source data, which have a greater density of medical decision-making knowledge. Secondly, we filtered the text in the chapters based on triggers and templates designed by medical experts to obtain text fragments containing knowledge of the medical decision process.

Our annotation team consisted of four annotators and two medical experts, all of whom received at least two hours of detailed and formal instruction in the principles of annotation. We use multiple rounds of annotation to annotate text fragments. Each text fragments was annotated independently by two annotators, and in cases of inconsistency and uncertainty, the final result was determined by expert discussion. Furthermore, we calculate the Cohen's Kappa [3] to measure the agreements between two annotators. The result of triplet annotation is 0.83, which indicates a high degree of consistency; the result of MDT annotation is 0.37, which indicates a degree of consistency.

4.2 Data Statistics

Table 1. Statistics of the medical decision tree in Text2DT dataset.

Tree_Depth	Amount	Proportion
2	134	26.80%
3	300	60.00%
4	64	12.80%
5	2	0.40%

Table 1 reports the statistics of the tree depth in the Text2DT dataset. There are 500 text-tree pairs in the Text2DT dataset; the decision tree depth is 2 to 5, the average number of nodes per tree is 3.76, and the average number of triplets per tree is 6.46. There are 1896 nodes in the dataset, including 934 decision nodes, 962 conditional nodes, 476 "or" nodes, 367 "and" nodes, and 1053 "null" nodes.

Table 2 reports the statistics of the decision tree structures in the Text2DT dataset (using the pre-sequence of nodes to represent the tree structure while ignoring triplets and logical relations logical relationship between triplets in the nodes). There are 7 tree structures in the Text2DT dataset. "◊□◊□□" is the most dominant tree structure, accounting for 50.60% of the total. In contrast, "◊◊□□◊□□" and "◊□◊□◊□◊□□" account for the least in the dataset, both accounting for 0.40%.

Table 3 reports the statistics of the triplet relations in the Text2DT dataset. Text2DT dataset has 6 relationships, where the relationship "forbidden_drug"

Table 2. Statistics of the decision tree structure in Text2DT dataset (using the pre-sequence of nodes to represent the tree structure).

Tree_structure	Amount	Proportion
◊□◊□□	253	50.60%
◊□□	134	26.80%
◊◊□□□	47	9.40%
◊□◊□◊□□	45	9.00%
◊◊□◊□□□	17	3.40%
◊◊□□◊□□	2	0.40%
◊□◊□◊□◊□□	2	0.40%

Table 3. Statistics of the triplet relations in Text2DT dataset.

Relation_Name	Amount	Proportion
clinical_feature	1374	42.51%
therapeutic_drug	910	28.15%
medical_option	561	17.36%
usage_or_dosage	222	6.87%
forbidden_drug	83	2.57%
basic_information	82	2.54%

only accounts for 2.57% percent of the total number of triplets, so the dataset exhibits long-tailed distributions. It should be noted that the triplet extraction in Text2DT has the problem of SingleEntityOverlap (SEO), i.e., triplets in medical text share a single entity.

4.3 Manual Evaluation of Medical Decision Trees

To evaluate the quality of the annotated medical decision tree and whether it can help make medical decisions, we invited 10 medical practitioners and 10 people without a medical background to complete the following two evaluation tasks: 1) We observed the subjects' performance (accuracy and time spent) in answering medical decision problems of similar difficulty under different settings (with medical texts or decision trees as a reference). 2) We asked subjects to evaluate the ability of medical texts and decision trees to represent the medical decision process (completeness, readability, helpfulness).

Most of the subjects could answer the decision-making questions more accurately or faster with the help of the MDTs and thought that our annotated MDTs are more readable and helpful for understanding the knowledge of the medical decision process while providing a comprehensive representation of decision knowledge in medical texts. This demonstrates the quality of our annotation and the strength of the decision tree in terms of expressive power. Besides, we provide a detailed manual evaluation of MDT in Appendix A.

5 Participating Teams and Methods

5.1 Participating Teams

This shared task is held in CHIP-2022 Conference as Shared Task 3. We use E-mails to release the datasets, collect participants' registrations, and receive the submissions of the participating teams. In total, 8 teams participated in the Text2DT shared task and submitted 13 individual runs. We have provided the team names, affiliations in Table 4. 5 teams are from industry and 3 teams are from universities or research institutions.

Table 4. All the participating teams.

Team name	Affiliation	#submission	Rank
WinHealth	WinHealth Technology, Co.,Ltd	1	1
Xitong God With Me	Wuhan Research Center, Iflytek Co.,Ltd	3	2
1mdata	Beijing Yiming Tech	2	3
Yongzhe Wujiang	Zhejiang University	1	4
Chuyi Shier Niansan	Data Ark	3	5
Chuangjie	Zhejiang Chuangjie Co., Ltd	1	1
Dadadada	Zhongyuan Institute of Technology	1	7
capybara	Dalian University of Technology	1	8

5.2 Test Results

We have provided the official results for the Text2DT task and baseline models in Table 5. We rank the submissions based on the Tree_Acc score. Team *WinHealth* achieved the first rank with 55.00% Tree_Acc score and also reported the highest Triplet_F1 score (94.39%) and DP_F1 score (69.27%). We observe that the top-3 teams achieved high performances for triple extractions. The main differences of performances are reflected in the DP_F1 score, which reflect the submitted systems' ability to reconstruct the decision trees.

Table 5. The official test results of the Text2DT 2022 shared task.

Team name	Rank	Tree_Acc	Triplet_F1	DP_F1	Edit_DT	Node_F1
WinHealth	1	0.5500	0.9439	0.6927	2.5700	0.8531
系统之神与我同在	2	0.5400	0.9279	0.6868	2.7200	0.8303
医鸣科技	3	0.3700	0.9019	0.5271	5.4100	0.7480
勇者无疆	4	0.3200	0.8992	0.4742	5.8500	0.7156
初一十二廿三	5	0.2900	0.8857	0.4710	5.6900	0.6631
创联网捷	1	0.2700	0.8670	0.4355	5.4700	0.6702
大大大大	7	0.2100	0.8537	0.3873	6.9400	0.5897
capybara	8	0.1900	0.7183	0.3215	7.1500	0.5688

5.3 Methods

In this subsection, we will analyze the methods adopted by the top ranked teams, especially the top-3 teams ("WinHealth", "系统之神与我同在", "医鸣科技"), and summarize our findings.

Pre-trained Backbones. Almost all the teams fine-tune Chinese pre-trained language models (CPLMs) to obtain high-quality contextualized sentence representations. As demonstrated in [10,12,21,34,36,39], although pre-trained on open-domain corpus, the pre-trained models are effective in modeling the semantics in medical related tasks. There are also work on developing domain-specific pre-trained models [9,30,33]. Pre-trained on a corpus that is similar to the downstream tasks, the domain-specific pre-trained models can usually achieve good performances on in-domain downstream tasks. In this task, the top-3 ranked teams have employed many different pre-trained models: (1) Chinese RoBERTa model[1]; (2) RoFORMer-v2[2]; (3) ERNIE-Health[3]; (4) MacBERT [4]; (5) Chinese PERT [5]; (6) Chinese UIE model [14].

Methods for Triple Extraction. Triple extraction is of central importance for this task, since all the nodes of the decision trees consist of triples. Traditionally, the extraction of triples are divided into two steps, entity extraction [26,35] and relation classification of entity pairs [31,38]. This pipeline method requires two independent models. Team "系统之神与我同在" adopt this pipeline strategy. The entity recognition model is BERT+CRF, and his relation classification model is implemented with UIE [14], a generation based method for information extraction. The pipeline methods are pointed out to be inefficient and prone to error propagation [22,32,37]. Recently, many methods that complete the two tasks in a single forward step inside a single are developed. Team "WinHealth" and "医鸣科技" both implemented GlobalPointer [20], which is a simple yet effective modification to the Biaffine model [6]. Team "WinHealth" also tried to apply more recent work like Partition Filter Network [27], which divides the encoding neurons into different partitions, thus explicitly modeling the interactions between the entity modeling and relation modeling process.

Methods for Tree Reconstruction. Although one can achieve high precision on the triple extraction process, the most difficult step of our task is the reconstruction of the decision trees, i.e., organizing the triples in a logic way to reflect the decision processes of medical professionals. To combine the triples into nodes in the tree, Team "医鸣科技" applies the Biaffine model to classifier the relations among triples ("and", "or", or "none" relation). Team "系统之神与我同在" mines patterns in the contexts and use key phrases to determine the relations among triples. Then they design heuristic rules to organize nodes into complete trees. Team "WinHealth" develops a multi-turn question answering system to determine how to organize the triples into nodes.

[1] https://huggingface.co/hfl/chinese-roberta-wwm-ext.
[2] https://github.com/ZhuiyiTechnology/roformer-v2.
[3] https://github.com/PaddlePaddle/PaddleNLP/tree/develop/model_zoo/ernie-health.

Other Training Techniques. Besides the above methods, the top teams also apply many different model training techniques. 3 teams employs R-Drop [13], which is to feed the samples twice to the networks with different dropout masks, and regularizes the distances between the two predicted distributions. Some teams find that fine-tuning with the masked language modeling (MLM) task [7,40] is helpful for boosting the downstream task performances. Data augmentations are widely applied, since our annotation data has relative small sample sizes.

By analyzing the top solutions, we can reform the following findings:

- The pre-trained backbones are essential to obtain high accuracy for tasks of limited samples sizes like our task.
- Recent advances in triple extraction can be transferred to our task to train better triple extraction models.
- Currently, the tree re-construction steps can be solved by heuristic rules, but we can also apply models to facilitate the process. In the future, we should improve the shared task by annotating more complex decision trees of different structures.

6 Conclusion

In this article, we review the data construction process and give a detailed introduction of our Text2DT shared task. Automatic evaluation and manual evaluation methods are discussed. Then we present the participating teams and test results of the shared task. Finally, we analyze the methodologies of the top performing teams. The solutions to our novel task relies heavily on the pre-trained models and the triple extraction methods.

Acknowledgements. This work was supported by NSFC grants (No. 61972155 and 62136002) and National Key R&D Program of China (No. 2021YFC3340700), and Shanghai Trusted Industry Internet Software Collaborative Innovation Center.

A Manual Evaluation of Annotated MDTs

The detail of our manual evaluation of medical decision trees are as follows:

1. We observed the subjects' performance on medical decision problems of similar difficulty under medical texts and MDTs. Specifically, subjects will answer three sets of medical decision questions, each group providing texts or decision trees containing the medical knowledge needed to answer the medical decision question. We observe their accuracy and time spent answering the decision question. Each set of questions is randomly selected from the question pool and is guaranteed to be of similar difficulty.
2. We invited subjects to rate medical texts and MDTs in terms of readability, completeness, and helpfulness. Specifically, we randomly selected five medical texts and MDTs expressing the same knowledge. We asked subjects to score

(0–3) them in terms of whether they were clear and easy to understand (readability), whether they were comprehensive and detailed (completeness), and whether they were helpful in understanding or studying medical knowledge (helpfulness).

Table 6. Results of manual evaluation of annotated MDTs. The results in the first field are for subjects without medical background, and the results in the second field are for medical practitioners. **A** represents the average accuracy of answering the medical decision questions. **T** represents the average seconds spent answering the medical decision questions. **R**, **C**, and **H** represent the readability, completeness, and helpfulness average scores.

	A	T	R	C	H
Text	0.64	31.5	2.26	2.70	2.33
DT	0.86	25.4	2.74	2.72	2.62
Text	0.94	21.6	2.50	2.74	2.68
DT	0.94	18.4	2.66	2.62	2.76

The results of the manual evaluation are shown in Table 6. We can draw the following conclusions:

For subjects without medical background, the medical decision tree helped them make more correct decisions in less time compared with the medical text and gained the highest scores for readability, completeness, and helpfulness. Theoretically, the completeness of the medical text should be better than the medical decision tree. Still, due to the poor readability of the medical text, the subjects may not have gained complete access to the knowledge contained in the medical text.

For medical practitioners, the medical decision tree group achieved the same accuracy on the medical decision questions as the medical text group, but the former took less time. The medical decision trees gained the highest readability and helpfulness scores and slightly lower completeness than the medical texts. The results demonstrate that the medical decision tree can help people make treatment decisions faster and better and can model medical decision knowledge clearly and intuitively, which can help readers better understand medical decision knowledge.

References

1. H.Z.L.L.: Overview of technology evaluation dataset for medical multimodal information extraction. J. Med. Inform. **43**(12), 2–5+22 (2022)
2. W.L.Z.W.: Text2dt: decision rule extraction technology for clinical medical text. J. Med Inform. **43**(12), 16–22 (2022)

3. Cohen, J.: A coefficient of agreement for nominal scales. Educ. Psychol. Measur. **20**(1), 37–46 (1960)
4. Cui, Y., Che, W., Liu, T., Qin, B., Wang, S., Hu, G.: Revisiting pre-trained models for Chinese natural language processing. In: Findings of the Association for Computational Linguistics: EMNLP 2020, pp. 657–668. Association for Computational Linguistics, Online (November 2020). https://doi.org/10.18653/v1/2020.findings-emnlp.58, https://aclanthology.org/2020.findings-emnlp.58
5. Cui, Y., Yang, Z., Liu, T.: Pert: Pre-training BERT with permuted language model. ArXiv abs/2203.06906 (2022)
6. Dozat, T., Manning, C.D.: Deep biaffine attention for neural dependency parsing. ArXiv abs/1611.01734 (2016)
7. Gao, T., Yao, X., Chen, D.: SimcSE: simple contrastive learning of sentence embeddings. ArXiv abs/2104.08821 (2021)
8. Grosan, C., Abraham, A.: Rule-based expert systems. In: ,Intelligent Systems Reference Library, vol. 17. Springer, Berlin pp. 149–185. Springer, Cham (2011). https://doi.org/10.1007/978-3-642-21004-4_7
9. Gu, Y., Tinn, R., Cheng, H., Lucas, M.R., Usuyama, N., Liu, X., Naumann, T., Gao, J., Poon, H.: Domain-specific language model pretraining for biomedical natural language processing. ACM Trans. Comput. Healthc. **3**, 1–23 (2020)
10. Guo, Z., Ni, Y., Wang, K., Zhu, W., Xie, G.T.: Global attention decoder for Chinese spelling error correction. In: Findings (2021)
11. Jiang, T., Zhao, T., Qin, B., Liu, T., Chawla, N.V., Jiang, M.: The role of: a novel scientific knowledge graph representation and construction model. In: Teredesai, A., Kumar, V., Li, Y., Rosales, R., Terzi, E., Karypis, G. (eds.) Proceedings of the 25th ACM SIGKDD International Conference on Knowledge Discovery & Data Mining, KDD 2019, Anchorage, AK, USA, August 4-8, 2019. pp. 1634–1642. ACM (2019). https://doi.org/10.1145/3292500.3330942, https://doi.org/10.1145/3292500.3330942
12. Li, X., et al.: Pingan smart health and SJTU at COIN - shared task: utilizing pre-trained language models and common-sense knowledge in machine reading tasks. In: Proceedings of the First Workshop on Commonsense Inference in Natural Language Processing. pp. 93–98. Association for Computational Linguistics, Hong Kong, China (November 2019). https://doi.org/10.18653/v1/D19-6011, https://aclanthology.org/D19-6011
13. Liang, X., et al.: R-drop: Regularized dropout for neural networks. ArXiv abs/2106.14448 (2021)
14. Lu, Y., et al.: Unified structure generation for universal information extraction. In: Annual Meeting of the Association for Computational Linguistics (2022)
15. Machado, A., Maran, V., Augustin, I., Wives, L.K., de Oliveira, J.P.M.: Reactive, proactive, and extensible situation-awareness in ambient assisted living. Expert Syst. Appl. **76**, 21–35 (2017)
16. Marcinkiewicz, M.A.: Building a large annotated corpus of English: The PENN treebank. Comput. Ling., **19**(2), 313–330 (1994)
17. Nohria, R.: Medical expert system-a comprehensive review. Int. J. Comput. Appl. **130**(7), 44–50 (2015)
18. Saibene, A., Assale, M., Giltri, M.: Expert systems: Definitions, advantages and issues in medical field applications. Expert Syst. Appl. **177**, 114900 (2021)
19. Shortliffe, E.H., Sepúlveda, M.J.: Clinical decision support in the era of artificial intelligence. JAMA **320**(21), 2199–2200 (2018)
20. Su, J., et al.: Global pointer: Novel efficient span-based approach for named entity recognition. ArXiv abs/2208.03054 (2022)

21. Sun, H., et al.: Medical knowledge graph to enhance fraud, waste, and abuse detection on claim data: model development and performance evaluation. JMIR Med. Inform **8** (2020)
22. Sun, T., et al.: A simple hash-based early exiting approach for language understanding and generation. ArXiv abs/2203.01670 (2022)
23. Tsumoto, S.: Automated extraction of medical expert system rules from clinical databases based on rough set theory. Inf. Sci. **112**(1–4), 67–84 (1998)
24. Uzuner, Ö., Solti, I., Cadag, E.: Extracting medication information from clinical text. J. Am. Med. Inform. Assoc. **17**(5), 514–518 (2010)
25. Wang, Y., Liu, X., Shi, S.: Deep neural solver for math word problems. In: Palmer, M., Hwa, R., Riedel, S. (eds.) Proceedings of the 2017 Conference on Empirical Methods in Natural Language Processing, EMNLP 2017, Copenhagen, Denmark, September 9-11, 2017. pp. 845–854. Association for Computational Linguistics (2017). https://doi.org/10.18653/v1/d17-1088, https://doi.org/10.18653/v1/d17-1088
26. Wen, C., Chen, T., Jia, X., Zhu, J.: Medical named entity recognition from unlabelled medical records based on pre-trained language models and domain dictionary. Data Intell. **3**(3), 402–417 (09 2021). https://doi.org/10.1162/dint_a_00105, https://doi.org/10.1162/dint_a_00105
27. Yan, Z., Zhang, C., Fu, J., Zhang, Q., Wei, Z.: A partition filter network for joint entity and relation extraction. In: Conference on Empirical Methods in Natural Language Processing (2021)
28. Yu, T., et al.: Spider: a large-scale human-labeled dataset for complex and cross-domain semantic parsing and text-to-SQL task. In: Riloff, E., Chiang, D., Hockenmaier, J., Tsujii, J. (eds.) Proceedings of the 2018 Conference on Empirical Methods in Natural Language Processing, Brussels, Belgium, October 31 - November 4, 2018. pp. 3911–3921. Association for Computational Linguistics (2018). https://doi.org/10.18653/v1/d18-1425, https://doi.org/10.18653/v1/d18-1425
29. Zhang, N., et al.: CBLUE: A Chinese biomedical language understanding evaluation benchmark. In: Muresan, S., Nakov, P., Villavicencio, A. (eds.) Proceedings of the 60th Annual Meeting of the Association for Computational Linguistics (Volume 1: Long Papers), ACL 2022, Dublin, Ireland, May 22-27, 2022. pp. 7888–7915. Association for Computational Linguistics (2022). https://doi.org/10.18653/v1/2022.acl-long.544, https://doi.org/10.18653/v1/2022.acl-long.544
30. Zhang, Z., Zhu, W., Zhang, J., Wang, P., Jin, R., Chung, pCEE-BERT: Accelerating BERT inference via patient and confident early exiting. In: NAACL-HLT (2022)
31. Zhu, W.: AutoRC: Improving BERT based relation classification models via architecture search. In: Proceedings of the 59th Annual Meeting of the Association for Computational Linguistics and the 11th International Joint Conference on Natural Language Processing: Student Research Workshop. pp. 33–43. Association for Computational Linguistics, Online (Aug 2021). https://doi.org/10.18653/v1/2021.acl-srw.4, https://aclanthology.org/2021.acl-srw.4
32. Zhu, W.: LeeBERT: Learned early exit for bert with cross-level optimization. In: Annual Meeting of the Association for Computational Linguistics (2021)
33. Zhu, W.: MVP-BERT: Multi-vocab pre-training for Chinese BERT. In: Proceedings of the 59th Annual Meeting of the Association for Computational Linguistics and the 11th International Joint Conference on Natural Language Processing: Student Research Workshop. pp. 260–269. Association for Computational Linguistics, Online (Aug 2021). https://doi.org/10.18653/v1/2021.acl-srw.27, https://aclanthology.org/2021.acl-srw.27

34. Zhu, W., et al.: paht_nlp @ MEDIQA 2021: multi-grained query focused multi-answer summarization. In: Proceedings of the 20th Workshop on Biomedical Language Processing. pp. 96–102. Association for Computational Linguistics, Online (Jun 2021). https://doi.org/10.18653/v1/2021.bionlp-1.10, https://aclanthology.org/2021.bionlp-1.10
35. Zhu, W., Ni, Y., Wang, X., Xie, G.: Discovering better model architectures for medical query understanding. In: Proceedings of the 2021 Conference of the North American Chapter of the Association for Computational Linguistics: Human Language Technologies: Industry Papers. pp. 230–237. Association for Computational Linguistics, Online (June 2021). https://doi.org/10.18653/v1/2021.naacl-industry.29, https://aclanthology.org/2021.naacl-industry.29
36. Zhu, W., Ni, Y., Xie, G., Zhou, X., Chen, C.: The DR-KGQA system for automatically answering medication related questions in Chinese. In: 2019 IEEE International Conference on Healthcare Informatics (ICHI), pp. 1–6 (2019). https://doi.org/10.1109/ICHI.2019.8904496
37. Zhu, W., Wang, X., Ni, Y., Xie, G.T.: GAML-BERT: Improving bert early exiting by gradient aligned mutual learning. In: Conference on Empirical Methods in Natural Language Processing (2021)
38. Zhu, W., Wang, X., Qiu, X., Ni, Y., Xie, G.T.: Autotrans: automating transformer design via reinforced architecture search. ArXiv abs/2009.02070 (2020)
39. Zhu, W., et al.: PANLP at MEDIQA 2019: pre-trained language models, transfer learning and knowledge distillation. In: Proceedings of the 18th BioNLP Workshop and Shared Task, pp. 380–388. Association for Computational Linguistics, Florence, Italy (August 2019). https://doi.org/10.18653/v1/W19-5040, https://aclanthology.org/W19-5040
40. Zuo, Y., Zhu, W., Cai, G.: Continually detection, rapidly react: Unseen rumors detection based on continual prompt-tuning. In: COLING (2022)

Medical Decision Tree Extraction: A Prompt Based Dual Contrastive Learning Method

Yiwen Jiang[1(✉)], Hao Yu[2], and Xingyue Fu[1]

[1] Winning Health Technology Group Co., Ltd., Shanghai, China
j_yw@winning.com.cn, f.xy@winning.com.cn
[2] School of Information and Electrical Engineering, Shanghai Normal University, Shanghai, China
1000496946@smail.shnu.edu.cn

Abstract. The extraction of decision-making knowledge in the form of decision trees from unstructured textual knowledge sources is a novel research area within the field of information extraction. In this paper, we present an approach to extract medical decision trees from medical texts (aka. Text2DT) in the 8th China Health Information Processing Conference (CHIP 2022) Open Shared Task[1]. Text2DT task involves the construction of tree nodes using relation triples, which extends upon the foundation of the named entity recognition and relation extraction tasks. Compared to the fixed event schema typically defined in the event extraction task, the tree structure allows a more flexible and variable approach to representing information. To achieve this novel task, we propose a prompt based dual contrastive learning method. The experimental results demonstrate that the decision tree constructed by our model can achieve an accuracy of 55% (65% using the relaxed metric).
[1](http://www.cips-chip.org.cn/2022/eval3)

Keywords: decision tree extraction · prompt learning · contrastive learning

1 Introduction

Decision trees are a reliable and effective decision support tool that results in high classification accuracy (e.g., disease diagnosis) by using a tree-like structure of gathered knowledge. Medical decision trees are one of the cores of intelligent medical systems such as computer-assisted system of diagnosis and treatment [8]. To build medical decision trees, traditional methods rely on a large number of medical experts constructing them manually. Considering that many knowledge sources of clinical decision-making are stored in the form of unstructured text, such as Clinical Practice Guidelines and Medical Textbooks, exploring how to use natural language processing techniques to automatically extract medical decision trees at scale from these knowledge sources is a very promising research direction.

B. Tang et al. (Eds.): CHIP 2022, CCIS 1773, pp. 103–116, 2023.
https://doi.org/10.1007/978-981-99-4826-0_10

As part of the 8th China Health Information Processing Conference (CHIP 2022) Open Shared Task [15], a corpus named Text2DT [6,14] was developed as a benchmark dataset for the objective of studying how to extract medical decision trees from medical texts.

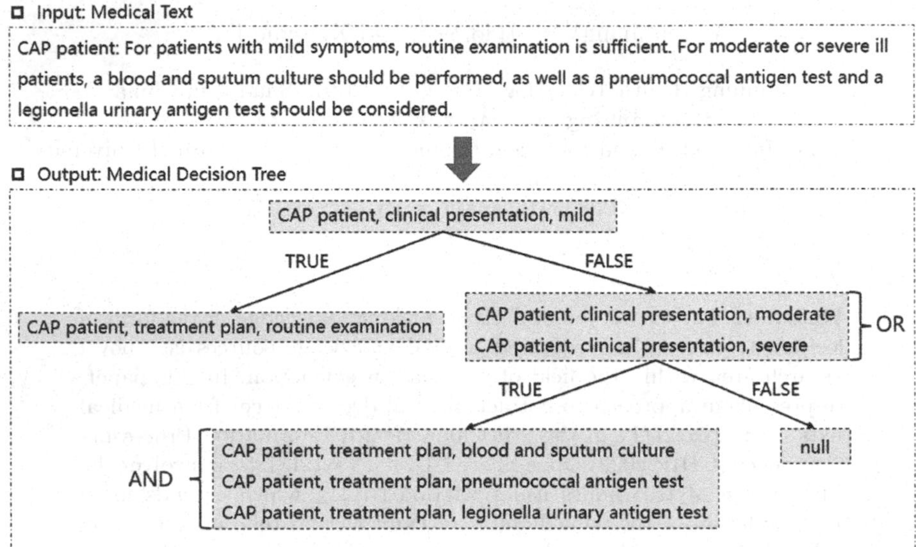

Fig. 1. An example about input and output of Text2DT task.

The process of clinical diagnosis and treatment can be conceptualized as a decision tree, as it involves making successive judgments based on various conditions and ultimately arriving at a decision. Figure 1 presents a visual representation of the input and output of the Text2DT task, showing an example of what a decision tree may look like. A medical decision tree is a binary tree structure and is composed of condition nodes and decision nodes. As illustrated in Fig. 1, condition nodes, represented by boxes with a light orange background, represent branch points in the tree where a judgment needs to be made. Decision nodes, represented by boxes with a light blue background, are always leaf nodes by definition and demonstrate the path taken based on the outcome of one or more condition nodes. The left child of a condition node indicates that the current condition is satisfied, while the right is not. To ensure the preorder sequence of a binary tree can uniquely determine its shape, we can add an empty node denoted by null, whenever the next judgment or decision of a certain condition node is not specified in the input text. The components that jointly determine each node in the decision tree include the type of node (i.e., condition or decision), as well as one or more triples represented as *(subject, relation, object)*, which are commonly defined in relation extraction tasks. In addition, multiple triples within a single node need to be related through logical operators (e.g.,

AND, OR). When there is only one triple or nothing in a node, the logical relation is absent. In Fig. 1, each box represents a node, and each row within the box represents a relation triple.

Text2DT can be considered as a novel subfield within the realm of information extraction, which traditionally includes tasks such as named entity recognition (NER), relation extraction (RE), and event extraction. The Text2DT task involves the construction of tree nodes using relation triples, which extends upon the foundation of the NER and RE task, as well as requires the classification of logical relations among triples. Event extraction often requires a pre-defined fixed schema for the identification of trigger words, argument roles, etc., while Text2DT involves tree structures that allow for a more flexible and variable approach in representing information in text. The key challenges in the Text2DT task involve the integration of multiple relation triples into individual nodes and the subsequent connection of these nodes into a decision tree structure, both of which make Text2DT task more complicated.

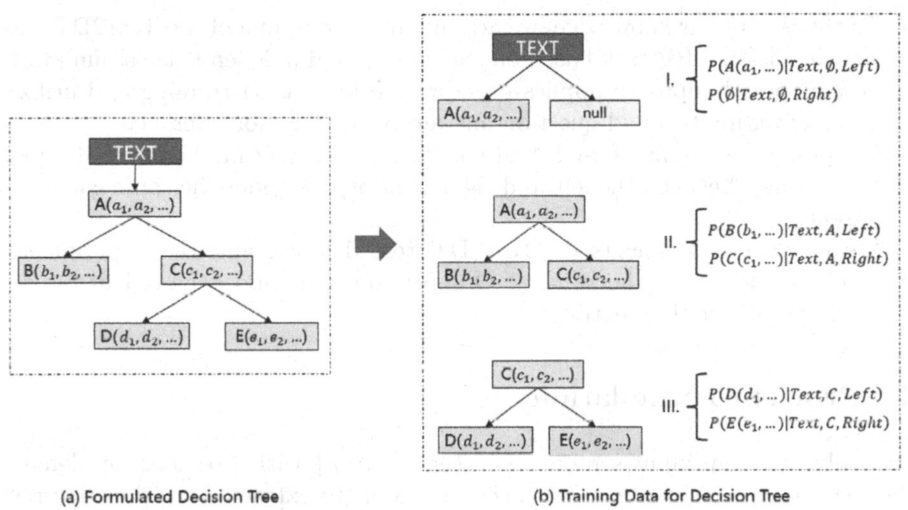

Fig. 2. Formulated Decision Tree and its training data.

In this paper, we propose a novel method to achieve Text2DT task. Inspired by the decision tree's inference process, which involves making successive judgments on condition nodes, we assume that each node in the tree only depends on its parent node and is independent on other nodes. With this assumption, we reformulate the problem of Text2DT as a conditional RE problem, in which each condition node serves as a condition (aka. prompt) for extracting relation triples from text, and the extraction result is the two children of the condition node. Figure 2(a) formulates the decision tree depicted in Fig. 1, in which the nodes are denoted by capital letters (e.g., A, B, etc.) and the i-th triple within a given node X is represented by x_i. During training, we follow the assumption of $P(X(x_1, x_2, \ldots) | Text, Condition, Operator)$, where $X \in \{A, B, \ldots\}$ is the target node for extraction in tree, $Text$ is the input sequence, $Condition$ is a prompt for extraction i.e., the parent node of X and $Operator \in \{Left, Right\}$ is applied to distinguish whether X is a left node or a right node. As shown in Fig. 2(b), for a decision tree with n condition nodes, it will generate $2 \times (n + 1)$ training data, where 1 represents the root node of the tree. To align the input for batch training, we suppose the condition for the extraction of root node is an empty set. The root node is then assigned as the left child, while the right child remains unoccupied. During the training phase, we utilize prompt learning to achieve conditional RE, describing the condition in natural language as a prompt. About inference, we employ a multi-round question and answer approach that simulates the reasoning process of a decision tree, naturally generating the whole tree in a recursive manner. Additionally, as the input for extracting the left and right nodes only differs in the operator, we propose a dual contrastive learning (DualCL) method to increase the distance between different child nodes under the same condition. In summary, our contributions include:

1. To the best of our knowledge, we are the first one to model the Text2DT task as a conditional RE task based on the conditional independence assumption. Our proposed approach applies prompt learning during training and utilizes a recursive, multi-round question answering strategy for inference.
2. We propose a prompt based dual contrastive learning method to pull apart the distance between the left and right child nodes under the same condition parent.
3. We conduct experiments on Text2DT test dataset, and the experimental results demonstrate the validity. Our proposed method achieved first place on all five evaluation metrics.

2 Problem Formulation

Formally, given an input sentence $s = \{w_1, \ldots, w_L\}$ with L tokens, w_i denotes the i-th token in sequence s. Text2DT task aims to extract a decision tree represented by a preorder sequence, denoted as $DT = [N_1, \ldots, N_H]$ with H nodes. The i-th node $N_i = \{C/D, L(tri_1, \ldots, tri_n)\}$, where C/D denotes N_i is either a condition or a decision node, tri_j denotes j-th relation triple within the node and $L \in \{AND, OR, NULL\}$ is a logical operator representing the logical relation among multiple triples. When $n > 1$, $L \in \{AND, OR\}$, otherwise $L = NULL$. When the order of any two condition nodes in a decision tree can be interchanged, they are sorted according to the order in which their subject and object are mentioned in s. Additionally, since empty nodes are set, each condition node has two child nodes. These regulations ensure that the preorder sequence of the decision tree for each input text is uniquely determined.

3 Method

In this section, we present our prompt based dual contrastive learning model for Text2DT task. The model architecture is shown in Fig. 3 and consists of an encoder and a Global Pointer Network (GPN) [10]. The encoder is used to generate task-specific contextual representations for NER and RE tasks. We adopt token-pair tagging method and utilize GPN as a basic token-pair linking unit for the prediction of entities and relations within a tree node. The encoder is described in Sect. 3.1, while the details of GPN and its tagging method are provided in Sect. 3.2. Additionally, we model the Text2DT task as a conditional RE task. In Sect. 3.3, we describe how we utilize prompt learning to design the input sequence of the model. To pull apart the distance between the left and right child nodes under the same parent, we propose a dual contrastive learning (DualCL) method in Sect. 3.4. The training details of our model and multi-round question answering inference method are outlined in Sect. 3.5.

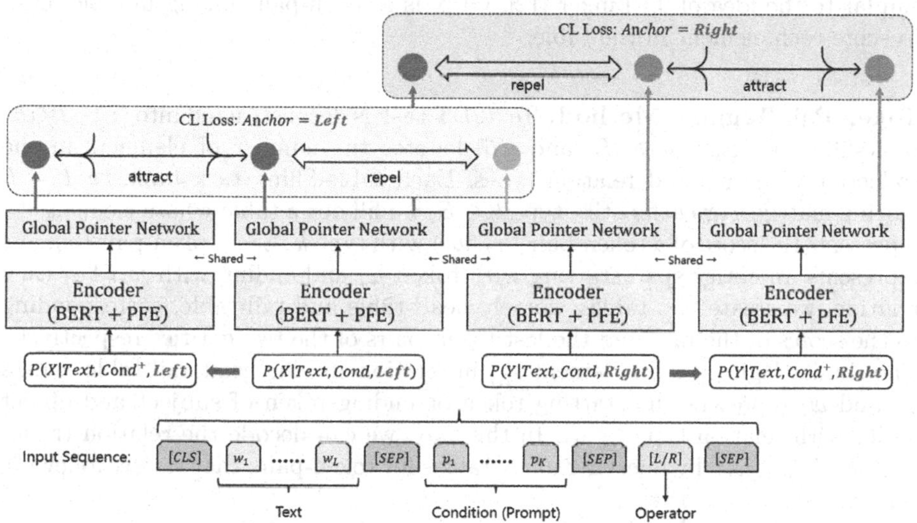

Fig. 3. The architecture of the proposed model.

3.1 Model Encoder

The encoder of the model consists of two parts, namely the BERT encoder [4] and Partition Filter Encoder (PFE) [13]. The BERT model is a multi-layer bidirectional Transformer encoder [11] based on self-attention mechanism. BERT is pre-trained on large-scale unannotated text datasets. The pre-trained model is then fine-turned to adapt to different downstream tasks, a process known as transfer learning. Given an input token sequence $s = \{w_1, \ldots, w_L\}$, after

12 stacked self-attention blocks, the output of BERT is a contextual representation sequence $H = h_1, \ldots, h_L$, and is then fed to PFE (a recurrent feature encoder) used to generate task-specific features. PFE aims to model balanced bi-directional interaction between NER and RE tasks. At each time step, this module follows two sub-steps: partition and filter. PFE first partitions each neuron into two task-specific partitions (namely entity partition and relation partition) to store intra-task information and one shared partition to store inter-task information that is valuable to both tasks, according to its contribution. And then different partitions are combined to filter task-irrelevant information to form the final features denoted by $H_n = h_1^n, \ldots, h_L^n$ and $H_r = h_1^r, \ldots, h_L^r$ for NER and RE tasks, respectively.

3.2 Global Pointer Network (GPN)

The purpose of this module is to jointly extract entities and relations in an input sequence. We formulate joint extraction as a type-specific table-filling problem, similar to the idea of TPLinker [12]. GPN is a token-pair linking module, used to score each element in the table.

Token Pair Tagging Method. Text2DT task is deconstructed into $|E|+2\times|R|$ table-filling tasks, where $|E|$ and $|R|$ denotes the number of elements in the collection of entity and relation types. Each table-filling task builds a $L \times L$ scoring matrix. For each entity type $k \in E$, we fill out a table whose element $e_{i,j}^k$ represents the score of a token-pair (w_i, w_j) with type k. Each token-pair (w_i, w_j) represents an entity span starting with token w_i and ending with w_j. For each relation, we create two tables, namely head-table and tail-table, corresponding to the scores of the first and the last token-pairs of the two entities respectively. The similar logic goes for element $r_{i,j}^l$ in relation-specific head/tail-table, where w_i and w_j represent the starting token or ending token of subject and object entity with relation type $l \in R$. In this way, we can decode the relation triples $\langle w_x, w_y, l, w_m, w_n \rangle$ by querying multi-tables for token-pairs that satisfy following conditions:

$$e_{x,y}^{k_s} \geq \lambda_e; e_{m,n}^{k_o} \geq \lambda_e; r_{x,m}^l \geq \lambda_r; r_{y,n}^l \geq \lambda_r \tag{1}$$

where λ_e and λ_r are the threshold for prediction, both are set to 0 by default. Additionally, it is necessary for the entity types of the subject k_s and object k_o in a triple to conform to the constraint requirements specified in the relation definition (see Table 1 for details).

Token Pair Linking Unit. Given task-specific features H_n or H_r, for each token-pair (w_i, w_j), two feedforward layers are used to map the head and tail token features h_i and h_j into low-dimensional vectors $q_{i,a}$ and $k_{j,a}$ as following:

$$\begin{aligned} q_{i,a} &= W_{q,a} h_i + b_{q,a} \\ k_{j,a} &= W_{k,a} h_j + b_{k,a} \end{aligned} \tag{2}$$

where $W_{q,a}$ and $W_{k,a}$ are parameter matrixes, as well as $b_{q,a}$ and $b_{k,a}$ are bias vectors for specific type α to be learned during training. Then, the score of the token-pair that leverages the relative positions through a multiplicative attention mechanism, is calculated by equation (3).

$$S_\alpha(i,j) = (R_i q_{i,a})^T (R_j k_{j,a}) \tag{3}$$

Rotary position embedding [9] is applied into the score calculation, which satisfies $R_i^T R_j = R_{j-1}$.

3.3 Prompt Learning

We utilize prompt learning for conditional RE. As shown in Fig. 3, the composition of the model input can be denoted as $P(X(x_1, x_2, \ldots) \mid Text, Condition, Operator)$, where $Text$ is the input sequence, $Condition$ is a prompt sequence describing the parent node Y of target node X to be extracted and $Operator$ is applied to distinguish whether X is a left node or a right node.

The tree node $Y = \{C, L(tri_1, \ldots, tri_n)\}$ is comprised of $n\,(n \geq 1)$ triples, and we employ the following steps to represent Y in natural language. Firstly, for any two triples $tri_x = (e_x^s, r_x, e_x^o)$ and $tri_y = (e_y^s, r_y, e_y^o)$, if $e_x^s = e_y^s$ and $r_x = r_y$, the triples are merged to reduce redundancy, e.g., the triple *(CAP patient, clinical presentation, moderate or severe)* generated in Fig. 1. Next, we develop natural language templates for each relation type and fill the slots within the template with the subject and object from the triple to generate a sentence. For example, the generated sentence from the aforementioned triple is "*The clinical presentation of a CAP patient is moderate or severe.*" The final prompt is generated by concatenating multiple sentences from multiple triples in the node, using conjunctions of AND/OR determined by their logical relation L to express connections.

We concatenate the given sentence s, prompt p and operator o with classification token $[CLS]$ and separator token $[SEP]$ in BERT as the input sequence: $[CLS]\ s\ [SEP]\ p\ [SEP]\ o\ [SEP]$. Operators $o \in \{[Left], [Right]\}$ are any of the two predefined special tokens to distinguish whether to extract the left or right child node based on p. In addition, to help the model locate the start position of each entity mentions in p, we change the position encoding of these entities to be exactly the same as those mentioned in s.

3.4 Dual Contrastive Learning (DualCL)

The purpose of DualCL is to improve model's capability of distinguish left and right nodes under the similar inputs. The left and right nodes represent the condition is satisfied and not satisfied, respectively. These two nodes are therefore can be considered as negative examples of each other. When implementing contrastive learning with one of the nodes as the anchor, the same approach can be applied to the other node. That is the reason why we refer to this method as DualCL.

Take the left node X as an example, we treat the input $P(X(x_1, \ldots, x_n)\,|Text, Condition, [Left])$ as an anchor. We start from introducing how the positive and negative examples are generated.

- **Positive examples.** Inspired by the idea of R-Drop [7], we feed the same input to the model twice, due to the dropout layers that randomly drop neurons, different sub-models will generate two different distributions, one of which we consider to be the positive example of the anchor.
- **Negative examples.** The corresponding right node $P(X(x_1, \ldots, x_n)\,|\,Text, Condition, [Right])$ with the same $Condition$ is regarded as a negative example.

We improve the models by contrasting relation-specific tables according to the head and tail token-pair representations. During the scoring process of token-pair (w_i, w_j) in GPN, the concatenation of vectors q_i and k_j is regarded as the feature representation denoted by $z_{ij} = [q_i; k_j]$. We treat each ground-truth relation-specific token-pair $(w_i, w_j) \in T_a$ as an anchor, where T_a represents any relation table. Then (w_i, w_j) is the golden answer to both T_a and the corresponding typed table in positive example T_p but not to that in negative example T_n. The contrastive learning loss is calculated as following:

$$CL\ loss = \frac{1}{T}\sum_{t=1}^{T}\frac{1}{B}\sum_{b=1}^{B}\frac{1}{N}\sum_{(i,j)\in t_a}^{N} -\log\frac{\exp(\frac{\varphi(z_{ijb}^{ta}, z_{ijb}^{tp})}{\tau})}{\exp(\frac{\varphi(z_{ijb}^{ta}, z_{ijb}^{tp})}{\tau}) + \exp(\frac{\varphi(z_{ijb}^{ta}, z_{ijb}^{tn})}{\tau})} \tag{4}$$

where $\varphi(u, v) = u^T v / \|u\| \cdot \|v\|$ is the cosine similarity between vectors u and v, $\tau > 0$ is a scalar temperature parameter, T is the number of relation tables, B is the batch size during training and N is the number of ground-truth token-pair in the table T_a. The final DualCL loss is calculated as the average of the left and right node losses, i.e.,

$$DualCL\ loss = \frac{1}{2}(Left\ CL\ loss + Right\ CL\ loss) \tag{5}$$

3.5 Training Details and Inference

Since the matrix of each typed table is extremely sparse, we use Class Imbalance Loss [10] during training. The total loss is calculated as the sum of losses from all task tables:

$$\log\left(1 + \sum_{(i,j)\in\Omega_{neg}^{a}} e^{-s_a^{(i,j)}}\right) + \log\left(1 + \sum_{(i,j)\in\Omega_{pos}^{a}} e^{s_a(i,j)}\right) \tag{6}$$

where (i, j) represent a token-pair (w_i, w_j), Ω_{neg}^{a} represents a collection of token-pairs that do not belong to type a, Ω_{pos}^{a} represents a collection of token-pairs whose entity type or relation type is a. In particular, formula (6) is a simplified version, when the threshold λ_e and λ_r are both 0. The final objective loss of our model is the sum of Class Imbalance Loss and DualCL loss.

During inference, we adopt a multi-round question and answer approach to naturally form a decision tree in a recursive manner. The first step is to initialize the root node R using $P(R|Text, \emptyset, [Left])$ input for the model. Secondly, the condition node R will serve as a new prompt to provide $P(X|Text, R, [Left])$ and $P(Y|Text, R, [Right])$ into the model, resulting in the generation of the left child X and right child Y. We will determine the next course of actions based on the type of the newly generated nodes. If the node is a condition node, we will repeat the second process mentioned above. If it is a decision node, we will terminate the current path. Through this recursive method, we can construct a complete decision tree. Additionally, we partition the relation types into either the condition partition or the decision partition (see Table 1 for details). The type of node depends on the partition with more extracted relation triples, while the result of the other partition is discarded. In the end, the logical operator of the node is determined by a heuristic algorithm.

4 Experiment

In this section, we provide data distribution details of Text2DT dataset, the leaderboard performance and an analysis of the effect of proposed method.

Table 1. Statistics for relation types in the Text2DT training set.

Relation Name	Subject Name	Object Name	Count	Partition
clinical presentation	patient	symptom	1106	condition
therapeutic drug	patient	drug	755	decision
treatment plan	patient	treatment	432	decision
dosage administration	drug	instruction	197	decision
basic information	patient	information	68	condition
contraindicated drug	patient	drug	65	decision
Overall	/	/	2623	/

4.1 Text2DT Dataset

The Text2DT dataset consists of 500 medical texts, with 400 used for model training and 100 for testing and final evaluation. As shown in Table 1, the dataset defines 6 types of relations. During the preprocessing phase, we further defined the partition of each relation and the entity types of the subject and object within each relation type (a total of 6 entity types such as patient and drug, etc.). The dataset is built on the following assumptions: (1) The medical texts included in the dataset are assumed to contain information relevant to decision-making processes, and there is no case where a decision tree cannot be extracted. (2) It is further assumed that each text in the dataset corresponds to a single decision tree, and there are no instances in which multiple decision trees can be extracted from a single text. Table 2 presents the distribution of various tree preorder sequences in the training dataset, where C and D indicate the condition and decision nodes respectively. The imbalanced distribution of tree structures does not impact the performance of our proposed model since the structural information of the entire tree is not involved during training.

The Text2DT task is evaluated using the following five metrics, sorted from relaxed to strict:

- **F1 score of triples.** The node is primarily composed of triples, and this metric evaluates all triples within the tree without considering any tree structure.
- **F1 score of nodes.** A decision tree is composed of multiple nodes, and this metric ignores the structure and decision paths of the tree, evaluating each node and requiring its type, logical operator and internal triples to be completely correct.
- **F1 score of decision paths.** A path from the root node to a leaf node is called a decision path, which represents the process of making a decision based on conditions. This metric is based on the decision path of the tree and requires that all nodes in the path are completely correct.
- **Edit distance of decision trees.** The edit distance in a decision tree refers to the minimum number of edit operations required to transform one tree into another. Tree edit operations include changing the type of a node; inserting or deleting triples; and modifying the logical relation among triples. The edit distance can measure the similarity of two trees and work as a more relaxed evaluation metric than the accuracy of decision trees.
- **Accuracy of decision trees.** The strictest evaluation metric in Text2DT task. The extracted decision tree is considered correct when it is completely consistent with the ground truth, including the tree structure, triples, and logical relations.

Table 2. Statistics for preorder sequence in the Text2DT training set.

Tree Preorder Sequence	Count
CDD	122
CDCDD	184
CDCDCDD	41
CCDDD	39
CCDCDDD	10
CDCDCDCDD	2
CCDDCDD	2
Overall	400

4.2 Experimental Setup

We randomly split the 400 labeled data into train and development datasets with the ratio of 4:1. The training set is utilized to learn model parameters, while the development set is utilized to select optimal hyperparameters. Since position information for each entity in the triples is not provided, we generated it using a heuristic algorithm and employed a five-fold cross-validation approach to apply ensemble learning to multiple models and evaluate the final performance on the test set.

4.3 Implementation and Hyperparameters

We tried different variants of the large-level BERT model, including RoBERTa [2], MacBERT [1] and PERT [3]. For all these pre-trained models, we employed the same set of following hyperparameters without any further fine-tuning. We used a batch size of 16 and employed the hierarchical learning rate in the training process with Adam optimizer [5], using a learning rate of $1e-5$ for pre-trained weights and $1e-4$ for other weights. We trained for at most 100 epochs with early stopping strategy based on the performance of development set. Training stops when the F1-score on the development set fails to improve for 12 consecutive epochs or the maximum number of epochs has been reached. To prevent overfitting and generate positive examples, dropout layers with a dropout rate of 0.1 are used. The dimensions of the hidden vectors for PFE and GPN are set to 512 and 128, respectively. We employed a combination of 15 models, each of which is trained using five-fold cross-validation on three different pretrained models, to make predictions at each recursive step, so the error propagation problem can be reduced during multiple rounds of question answering.

4.4 Results

Table 3 presents the results of different pre-trained models, with the average scores obtained in the development set through five-fold cross-validation. The large-level PERT model yields the highest performance, achieving micro-F1 score of 81.71%. where the F1 score is the evaluation metric for the conditional RE task, used to evaluate the triples within each node. It is more stringent compared to the final evaluation metric for triples defined in the Text2DT dataset.

Table 3. Model results in development set with different pre-trained models.

Model	Micro-F1 Score
$\text{RoBERT}_{\text{Large}}$	81.47
$\text{MacBERT}_{\text{Large}}$	80.70
$\text{PERT}_{\text{Large}}$	81.71

The results for final evaluation are summarized in Table 4. Our proposed method ranks first against all five evaluation metrics. Two evaluation methods are set up in the experiments, one of which takes the logical relations within the nodes into consideration, while the other ignores them. Our method performs best in terms of extracting triples, achieving an F1 score of 94.39%. The evaluation metric for nodes is most similar to that in the training process, however, the logical relations are not considered during training (a simple heuristic method is applied in post-processing), which results in a loss of 4.42% F1 score for the performance. The evaluation results of the decision paths well reflect how many decisions are correct when using the constructed tree for reasoning. Finally, the strictest standard indicates that 55% of the constructed tree is completely correct, and this number reaches 65% when ignoring logical relations. On average, only 2.57 edit operations are needed to modify the tree into the correct one.

Table 4. Evaluation results of five metrics in test set.

Method	Triple-F1	Node-F1	Path-F1	Tree-Acc	Tree-Edit
Consid.logic.rel	94.39	85.31	69.27	55.00	2.57
Ignore logic.rel		89.73	78.44	65.00	2.15

4.5 Ablation Study

To evaluate the validity of each component of our approach, we conducted ablation experiments using base-level RoBERTa on the development set. As illustrated in Table 5, incorporating PFE can enhance model's performance and DualCL is effective for the model, increasing the F1 score by 1.53%.

Table 5. Ablation study in development set.

Model	Micro-F1
$\text{RoBERT}_{\text{Base}}$	79.39
w/o PFE	76.98
w/o DualCL	77.86

5 Conclusion and Discussion

In this paper, we proposed a prompt based dual contrastive learning method for extracting medical decision tree from medical text. The Text2DT problem is reformulated as a conditional RE problem during training and a recursive multi-round question answering strategy is utilized for inference. Our experiments demonstrated that prompt learning and PFE can effectively achieve conditional RE, as well as DualCL method can further improve the model's performance. However, how to combine semantic information to determine the logical relation within each node is still an unsolved problem during training. Additionally, since current dataset is based on the two idealized assumptions, how to determine whether the text contains decision-making knowledge, and how to identify the number of decision trees in text are two crucial issues that cannot be overlooked in future work.

References

1. Cui, Y., Che, W., Liu, T., Qin, B., Wang, S., Hu, G.: Revisiting pre-trained models for Chinese natural language processing. In: Proceedings of the 2020 Conference on Empirical Methods in Natural Language Processing: Findings. pp. 657–668. Association for Computational Linguistics, Online (November 2020)
2. Cui, Y., Che, W., Liu, T., Qin, B., Yang, Z.: Pre-training with whole word masking for Chinese BERT. IEEE/ACM Trans. Audio Speech Lang. Proces. **29**, 3504–3514 (2021)
3. Cui, Y., Yang, Z., Liu, T.: PERT: pre-training BERT with permuted language model. arXiv preprint arXiv:2203.06906 (2022)
4. Devlin, J., Chang, M.W., Lee, K., Toutanova, K.: BERT: pre-training of Deep Bidirectional Transformers for Language Understanding. In: Proceedings of the 2019 Conference of the North American Chapter of the Association for Computational Linguistics: Human Language Technologies, Volume 1 (Long and Short Papers). pp. 4171–4186. Association for Computational Linguistics, Minneapolis, Minnesota (2019)
5. Kingma, D.P., Ba, J.: Adam: a Method for stochastic optimization. In: Bengio, Y., LeCun, Y. (eds.) 3rd International Conference on Learning Representations, ICLR 2015, San Diego, CA, USA, 7–9 May 2015, Conference Track Proceedings (2015)
6. Li, W., Zhu, W., Wang, X., Wu, Y., Ji, W., Tang, B.: Text2DT: decision rule extraction technology for clinical medical text. J. Med. Inform. **43**(12), 16–22 (2022)
7. Liang, X.., et al.: R-drop: Regularized dropout for neural networks. In: Advances in Neural Information Processing Systems. vol. 34, pp. 10890–10905. Curran Associates, Inc. (2021)
8. Podgorelec, V., Kokol, P., Stiglic, B., Rozman, I.: Decision trees: an overview and their use in medicine. J. Med. Syst. **26**(5), 445–463 (2002)
9. Su, J., Lu, Y., Pan, S., Wen, B., Liu, Y.: Roformer: enhanced transformer with rotary position embedding. arXiv preprint arXiv:2104.09864 (2021)
10. Su, J., et al.: Global pointer: novel efficient span-based approach for named entity recognition. arXiv preprint arXiv:2208.03054 (2022)
11. Vaswani, A., et al.: Attention is all you need. In: Advances in Neural Information Processing Systems. vol. 30. Curran Associates, Inc. (2017)

12. Wang, Y., Yu, B., Zhang, Y., Liu, T., Zhu, H., Sun, L.: TPLinker: single-stage joint extraction of entities and relations through token pair linking. In: Proceedings of the 28th International Conference on Computational Linguistics. pp. 1572–1582. International Committee on Computational Linguistics, Barcelona, Spain (Online) (December 2020)
13. Yan, Z., Zhang, C., Fu, J., Zhang, Q., Wei, Z.: A Partition filter network for joint entity and relation extraction. In: Proceedings of the 2021 Conference on Empirical Methods in Natural Language Processing. pp. 185–197. Association for Computational Linguistics, Online and Punta Cana, Dominican Republic (2021)
14. Zhu, W., Li, W., Wang, X.: Extracting decision trees from medical texts: an overview of the Text2DT track in CHIP 2022. In: Health Information Processing: 8th China Conference. CHIP 2022, pp. 21–23. Springer Nature Singapore, Hangzhou, China (October (2022)
15. Zong, H., et al.: Overview of technology evaluation dataset for medical multimodal information extraction. J. Med. Inform. **43**(12), 2–5 (2022)

An Automatic Construction Method of Diagnosis and Treatment Decision Tree Based on UIE and Logical Rules

Shiqi Zhen[1](✉) and Ruijie Wang[2]

[1] China University of Geosciencest, Wuhan 430000, Hubei, China
13476111882@163.com

[2] Wuhan University of Technology, Wuhan 430000, Hubei, China

Abstract. In traditional information extraction, entity relation triples are mainly extracted from text, and there is no further logical relationship between triples. Therefore, an information extraction model based on triple extraction and decision tree generation is proposed. The model first extracts the triples in the medical text through the UIE method, and then forms the triples into a binary tree according to the condition node and the decision node. The condition node represents the condition judgment that needs to be made, and the decision node represents the diagnosis and treatment decision that needs to be made. This decision can not only mine the core entities and relationships in the text, but also realize the connection of entity relationship information to form a complete decision process. The correct rate of decision tree construction has achieved good results, which proves that the model can effectively generate decision trees.

Keywords: Decision tree · Entity extraction · Relation extraction

1 Introduction

Information extraction aims to identify and construct user-specified information from unstructured text. Information extraction has a high degree of diversity due to different targets. Traditional named entity recognition and relation extraction play an important role in information extraction. Because the results of confidence extraction are structured, they can be easily applied to different fields, such as medical entity extraction. In the field of medicine, doctors need to focus on the patient in diagnosis, treatment and evaluation, highlight the causal relationship and the relationship between upper and lower positions in medicine, etc. There are a large number of medical questions and answers and a large number of causal relationship explanations in knowledge texts on the Internet, which are also of great value for medical search and diagnosis business while helping patients, From it, we can excavate and extract the medical causal relationship to build the causal relationship interpretation network, build the medical causal knowledge graph, and improve the ability to judge the logicality and interpretability of medical results.

At present, most relational extraction methods focus on the triples themselves, but ignore the logic between different triples, which results in its application in the medical

B. Tang et al. (Eds.): CHIP 2022, CCIS 1773, pp. 117–126, 2023.
https://doi.org/10.1007/978-981-99-4826-0_11

field has certain limitations, and knowledge cannot be maximized, which hinders the rapid development of information extraction in the medical field. As the core of intelligent medical systems such as auxiliary diagnosis and treatment system and medical teaching, the acquisition of diagnosis and treatment decision tree often depends on the manual construction of experts, which requires a lot of domain knowledge and is time-consuming and laborious. Therefore, it is of great significance to explore how to automatically extract the diagnosis and treatment decision tree (hereinafter referred to as Text2DT [1, 2]) from the diagnosis and treatment decision knowledge sources (clinical diagnosis and treatment guides, medical textbooks). Clinical diagnosis and treatment can be seen as a process of making judgments according to different conditions and then making different decisions. This clinical diagnosis and treatment process can be modeled as a clinical diagnosis and treatment decision tree. The clinical diagnosis and treatment decision tree is a tree structure composed of condition nodes and decision nodes. The condition nodes represent the condition judgments that need to be made, and the decision nodes represent the diagnosis and treatment decisions that need to be made. The diagnosis and treatment decision tree represents a simplified decision-making process, that is, making the next conditional judgment or decision according to the different results of conditional judgment. Once the decision is made, the diagnosis and treatment process is terminated. Therefore, we define the diagnosis and treatment decision tree as a binary tree composed of condition nodes and decision nodes, as shown in Fig. 1.

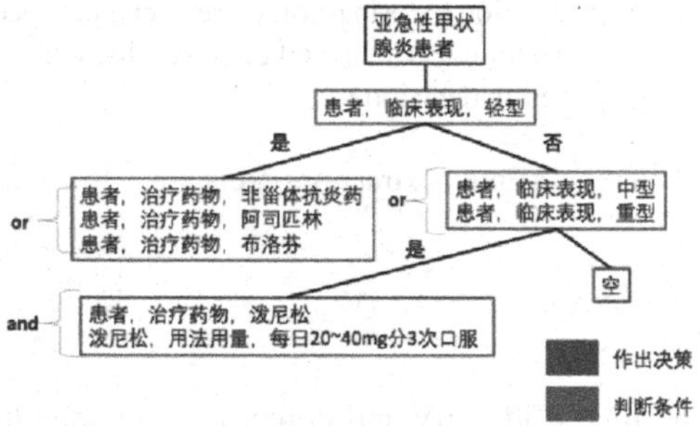

Fig. 1. Diagnosis and treatment decision tree.

As shown in Fig. 1, in the diagnosis and treatment decision binary tree, the non-leaf node is the condition node, and the leaf node is the decision node. For the condition node, when the condition judgment result is "Yes", it will go to the left sub-node for the next judgment or decision. When the condition judgment result is "No", it will go to the right sub-node for the next judgment or decision.Each node can be represented as $N = \{c/d, L(tri_1, \ldots\ldots, tri_n)\}$, where c/d indicates that the node is a condition/decision node; $tri_1, \ldots\ldots, tri_n$ represents n triples, that is, the contents of condition/decision nodes; L represents the logical relationship between multiple triples (or, and, when only one triple is empty). Note that if the next condition judgment or decision after a condition judgment result is "yes" or "no" is not expressed by the text semantics, an empty node is added to indicate that the next condition judgment and decision are unknown (that is, each condition node has two sub-nodes on the left and right side. If a node on one side does not exist in the text semantics, an empty node is added on this side). Therefore, each decision binary tree can be represented by the node's pre-order sequence.

2 Related Work

Information extraction (IE) is the task of extracting information (structured data) from text (unstructured data). For example, named entity recognition (NER) can recognize entities that appear in text. Relationship extraction (RE) identifies the relationship between entities. Event extraction (EE) finds events that occur in the text.

Researchers usually transform this task form into a natural language understanding problem. The latest methods of NER are based on the pre-training model BERT to perform the task. RE tasks have pipeline method and end-to-end method. The pipeline method divides tasks into NER and relationship classification, and executes two subtasks in order. The end-to-end rule jointly performs two subtasks. The latest EE method also uses BERT, and uses the pre-training model with tasks such as NER and RE.

Open information extraction is also an important task in information extraction. Its purpose is to extract information from text without relying on clearly defined patterns. However, whether it is NER, RE or EE, it extracts simple structured information, and there is no logical relationship between structured information.

Recently, Unified Relationship Extraction (UIE) defined all IE problems as seq2seq, that is, defined the transformation of structured input text into internal representation. The advantage of UIE is that it can use a single model to extract various structured information and achieve SOTA effect in multiple data sets. The disadvantage is that the structured definition is complex, and it is difficult to define non-NER, non-RE and non-EE extraction forms.

3 Diagnosis and Treatment Decision Tree Generation

The method in this paper firstly segments the text and uses UIE to extract the triples in the text. Then we classify the triples, that is, judge whether the triples are condition nodes or decision nodes, combine the triples of the same node type, and gradually generate a binary tree according to the order of text segmentation and the characteristics of different nodes. Finally, the logical relationship of the triad in the node is judged (AND or OR), and the diagnosis and treatment decision tree is finally generated. The system architecture is shown in Fig. 2.

3.1 Triple Extraction and Text Segmentation

3.1.1 Triple Extraction

UIE (Universal Information Extraction [3]): Yaojie Lu et al. proposed the universal information extraction unified framework UIE. It can generally model different information extraction tasks, adaptively generate target structures, and learn common IE capabilities from different knowledge sources. Specifically, UIE uniformly encodes different extraction structures through structured extraction language, adaptively generates target

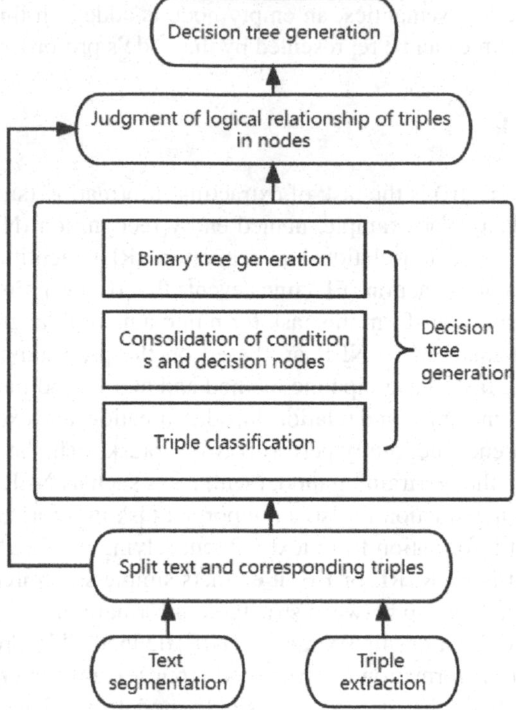

Fig. 2. System architecture of the model.

extraction through pattern-based prompt mechanism, and captures common IE capabilities through large-scale pre-trained text-to-structure model. UIE has achieved the most advanced performance in all supervised, low-resource and few-shot settings for a wide range of entities, relationships, events and emotion extraction tasks and their unification. Considering that the number of data sets in CHIP2022 is small and belongs to the few-shot category, we use UIE to complete the triple extraction to ensure the generalization of the results.

According to the observation data set, the head entities of "basic information", "clinical manifestation", "treatment plan", "therapeutic drugs" and "prohibited drugs" are the main patients, and the head entities of "usage and dosage" are a "therapeutic drug". Given an example sentence, for example, a patient with subacute thyroiditis@a medium-sized patient can be given prednisone 20–40 mg per day for 3 times. The "subacute thyroiditis patient" before the "@" sign is the main patient, and the "basic situation", "clinical manifestation", "treatment plan", "treatment drug" and "prohibited drug" are selected in turn. Take the "basic situation" as an example, and input it into the UIE: [CLS] basic situation [SEP] medium and severe patients can be given prednisone 20–40 mg minutes 3 times a day [SEP], The "basic information" is the prompt used to extract the "basic information" of the main patient, and the other triples of the main patient are extracted and so on. This example sentence can draw out the following triples of the main patient: ['subacute thyroid patient', 'clinical manifestation', 'medium'] and ['subacute thyroid patient', 'therapeutic drug', 'prednisone']. It can be found that the treatment drug of the main patient has been extracted, so a prompt of "usage and dosage" is constructed, with the paradigm of "usage and dosage of prednisone", which is input into UIE: [CLS] usage and dosage of prednisone [SEP] Medium-sized and severe patients can be given prednisone 20–40 mg/day for 3 times [SEP], and the triple group ['prednisone', 'usage and dosage', '20–40 mg/day for 3 times'] is obtained. The resulting triple will be placed in the node of the decision tree. Note that the triples here are with character subscripts and will be used for the next step.

3.1.2 Text Segmentation

In this step, the text is divided into segments according to the first-level separators ";" and ".", and then into clauses according to the second-level separators "," and ":". The extracted triples are matched according to the subscript index and clauses.

Take this sentence as an example: patients with subacute thyroiditis @ mild patients only need to use non-steroidal anti-inflammatory drugs, such as aspirin, ibuprofen, etc.; Medium-sized and severe patients can be given prednisone 20–40 mg daily for 3 times. According to the first-level separator, the main patient "patients with subacute thyroiditis" is not counted, and two segments are obtained: "light patients only need to use non-steroidal anti-inflammatory drugs, such as aspirin, ibuprofen, etc." and "medium and severe patients can be given prednisone 20 to 40 mg daily for three times". Then according to the second-level separator, the two sub-sentences of segment I are obtained: "light patients only need to use non-steroidal anti-inflammatory drugs" and "such as aspirin, ibuprofen, etc.", And a sub-sentence of segment 2, "Medium-sized and severe patients can be given prednisone 20–40 mg daily for 3 times" (i.e. segment 2 itself). Taking the triple group ['subacute thyroid patient', 'clinical manifestation', 'medium'] as an example, if the subscript of the tail entity "medium" is known to be [36, 37], then the clause "medium and severe patients can be given prednisone 20–40 mg daily for three times" can be matched, because the subscript range of this clause is [36, 59]. Therefore, triples are associated with clauses in this way. Now each clause has its corresponding triples.

3.2 Decision Tree Generation

3.2.1 Triple Classification

According to the data analysis results, the nodes corresponding to "basic situation" and "clinical manifestation" are condition nodes (defined as C nodes), and the nodes corresponding to "treatment scheme", "treatment drug", "prohibited drug" and "usage and dosage" are decision nodes (defined as D nodes).

3.2.2 Consolidation of Conditions and Decision Nodes

There are only two types of nodes in the decision tree, one is the condition node and the other is the decision node. Their contents are composed of one or more triples, which need to be put into the node.

Given example: patients with subacute thyroiditis @ mild patients only need to use non-steroidal anti-inflammatory drugs, such as aspirin, ibuprofen, etc.; Medium-sized and severe patients can be given prednisone 20–40 mg daily for 3 times. Through the previous steps, we can get the triples contained in each clause as follows:

"Light patients only need to use non-steroidal anti-inflammatory drugs" consists of three groups [['subacute thyroid patients',' clinical manifestations', 'light'], ['subacute thyroid patients',' therapeutic drugs', 'non-steroidal anti-inflammatory drugs']. The two triplets belong to condition node C and decision node D respectively, and [CD] is obtained;

"For example, aspirin, ibuprofen, etc." includes [['subacute thyroid patients',' therapeutic drugs', 'aspirin'], ['subacute thyroid patients',' therapeutic drugs', 'ibuprofen']]. Both triplets belong to decision node D, and [DD] is obtained;

"Medium-sized and severe patients can be given prednisone 20 to 40 mg per day for three times" includes [['subacute thyroid patients',' clinical manifestations', 'medium'], ['subacute thyroid patients',' clinical manifestations', 'severe'], ['subacute thyroid patients',' therapeutic drugs', 'prednisone'], ['prednisone', 'dosage', '20 to 40 mg per day for three times'], of which the first two triplets belong to condition node C, and the last two triplets belong to decision node D, Get [CCDD].

All nodes are [CD, DD|CCDD], where different segments are separated by "|" and different clauses are separated by ",". CC (or DD) in the same clause is combined into C (or D), so [CD, D|CD] is obtained. And C or D in the same segment are merged into the same node to get [C_1D_1|C_2D_2] four nodes. Take the above example sentence for example, C_1 is [['subacute thyroid patient', 'clinical manifestation', 'mild']; D_1 is [['subacute thyroid patients',' therapeutic drugs', 'non-steroidal anti-inflammatory drugs'], [' subacute thyroid patients', 'therapeutic drugs',' aspirin '], [' subacute thyroid patients', 'therapeutic drugs',' ibuprofen ']; C_2 is [['subacute thyroid patients',' clinical manifestations', 'moderate'], ['subacute thyroid patients',' clinical manifestations', 'severe']; D_2 is [['subacute thyroid patients',' therapeutic drugs', 'prednisone'], ['prednisone', 'usage and dosage', '20–40 mg/day, 3 times per day']. Therefore, several nodes and triples contained in nodes have been determined.

3.2.3 Binary Tree Generation

There are seven forms of decision tree in training dataset, as shown in Fig. 3.

By analyzing the above decision tree structure diagram, we find that the decision tree follows the basic rule of binary tree, that is, the condition node C must contain two sub-nodes. The sub-nodes may be the condition node C or the decision node D, but the leaf node (the node without sub-nodes) can only be the decision node D, that is, D has no sub-nodes.

Following this rule, we put nodes into the decision tree. Take the example sentence in the previous section for example. Now we have four nodes [C_1D_1|C_2D_2], which are divided into the following steps:

(1) Find the first condition node C, put it in the root node, and automatically generate left and right empty nodes to get [C1, empty, empty];
(2) The decision node D in the same segment as the condition node C is placed on the left node to get [C_1, D_1, empty];

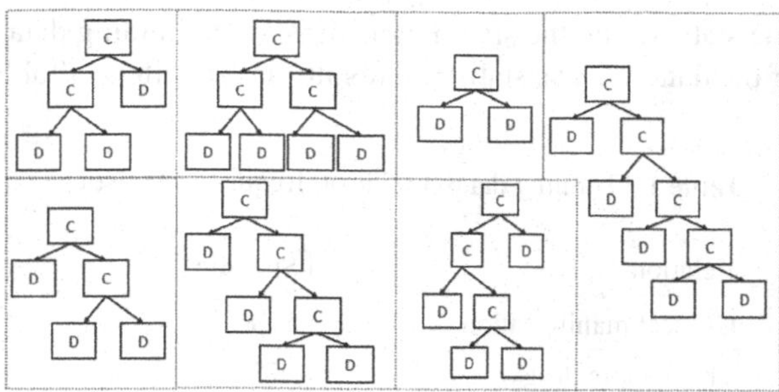

Fig. 3. Summary of decision tree structure.

(3) If the previous condition node C has a left node, the second condition node C will be placed on the right node; Otherwise, put the left node. So we get [C_1, D_1, C_2, empty, empty];

(4) The decision node D is placed on the left node by default, unless the turning word "but" appears. Therefore, [C_1, D_1, C_2, D_2, empty] is obtained, and the overall decision tree is shown in Fig. 1.

3.3 Judgment of Logical Relationship of Triples in Nodes

When there is only one triple in the node, the logical relationship is empty; However, when a node contains multiple triples, you need to determine whether the logical relationship between the multiple triples is "and" or "or".

Based on the segment, we judge the logical relationship according to the keywords appearing in the segment text: (1) the keywords of or: [or], [,, etc.], [may, such as]..., where [,, etc.] means "," and "etc." appear in the text at the same time; (2) Keywords of and: ['simultaneous',' joint ',' subsequent ',' combined ',' still needed ',' + ',' and ',' of '...]. It should be noted that the fragment text here is the text that intercepts the start and end positions of the triples in the fragment. Given example: patients with abnormal uterine bleeding @ tranexamic acid or non-steroidal anti-inflammatory drugs can be used for those who do not want to use sex hormone treatment or want to get pregnant as soon as possible. This sentence has only one segment, and the condition node contains two triplets: [abnormal uterine bleeding patient, basic situation, unwilling to use sexual hormone treatment] and [abnormal uterine bleeding patient, basic situation, want to pregnancy as soon as possible]. You can find the keywords "or" between the two tail entities "unwilling to use sexual hormone treatment" and "want to pregnancy as soon as possible" in the original text, so it is determined that the logical relationship of this node is "or". In this way, the logical relationship of triples in each node can be determined.

4 Experiment

4.1 Experimental Data

The data of this experiment was officially provided by CHIP2022, and the labeling data were all from the labeling of the published diagnosis and treatment guidelines and medical textbooks [4]. Training data: 300; Validation data: 100; Test data: 100.

We have made statistics on the six relationships in the training data to facilitate the understanding of the data set. The statistical results are as follows (Table 1).

Table 1. Training dataset relation frequency statistics.

Relation	Statistic
Clinical manifestation	1106
Therapeutic drugs	755
Treatment plan	432
Usage and dosage	197
Basic information	68
Prohibited drugs	65
Total	2623

The meaning of each relation is as follows: (1) Clinical manifestations: In order to avoid the long tail relationship and control the difficulty of the task, we call the clinical symptoms, physical signs and examination results of the patients "clinical manifestations"; (2) Therapeutic drugs: drugs with therapeutic and preventive effects that can improve or recover patients' diseases and keep them healthy are called "therapeutic drugs"; (3) Treatment plan: the treatment methods and suggestions other than drugs to make the patient better or recover are collectively referred to as "treatment plan"; (4) Usage and dosage: The usage ("oral", "intravenous", etc.) and dosage ("20–40 mg three times a day", etc.) of the drug are collectively referred to as "usage and dosage"; (5) Basic information: the patient's gender, age and intention are collectively referred to as "basic information"; (6) Prohibited drugs: drugs that are not recommended or prohibited in clinical practice are called "prohibited drugs".

4.2 Evaluating Indicators

Four evaluation indicators are designed in this experiment:

(1) F1 scores of triples extraction.
(2) Accuracy of the decision tree: the extracted decision tree is considered correct when it is completely consistent with the ground truth (tree structure, triple, logical relationship).
(3) F1 score of the decision path. We call the path from root node to leaf node to a decision path, which represents the process of making a decision based on conditional judgment. F1 score of decision path is a looser evaluation index than the accuracy of decision tree. For example, as shown in Fig. 1, there are two decision paths in this tree.
(4) Editing distance of the decision tree: similar to the editing distance of the string, the editing distance in the diagnosis and treatment decision tree is the minimum number of tree editing operations required to convert from one tree to another. Tree editing

operations include inserting and deleting nodes and changing the role of nodes; Insert and delete triples; And modify the logical relationship between triples. The editing distance can measure the similarity of two trees, as a more relaxed evaluation index than the accuracy of the decision tree. The editing distance of the following two trees is 5 (that is, the first tree needs to be changed into the second tree: 1. Add triplets (patients, clinical manifestations, heavy); 2. Add logical relationship or; 3 Modify the logical relationship or to and; 4. Delete the triad (patient, therapeutic drug, ibuprofen); 5. Add triplet (patient, treatment drug, prednisone).

4.3 Experimental Results

We fine-tune the model based on the Chinese UIE Basic (Base) version released by Baidu. The model has a total of 12 layers. The dimension of hidden variables in Transformer is 768. The number of attention heads in multi-head attention mechanism is 12. The total number of parameters exceeds 110M. Our final results in the four evaluation indicators are shown in Table 2, ranking second among all teams.

Table 2. Results of four experimental indicators.

F1 scores of triples extraction	92.79%
Accuracy of the decision tree	54%
F1 score of the decision path	68.68%
Editing distance of the decision tree	2.72%

5 Conclusion

The decision tree generation aims to automatically extract the diagnosis and treatment decision tree from the diagnosis and treatment decision knowledge sources (clinical diagnosis and treatment guides, medical textbooks, etc.).

This paper proposes an automatic construction method of diagnosis and treatment decision tree based on UIE and logical rules, which can automatically analyze the diagnosis and treatment text, extract the condition knowledge and decision knowledge contained in it, and automatically construct the diagnosis and treatment decision tree through the logical rules observed from the data set. The method in this paper avoids the complexity of manually constructing features. The accuracy rate of the evaluation data set of CHIP2022 evaluation three "extracting diagnosis and treatment decision tree from medical text" is 54%, ranking second among all teams, indicating the effectiveness of the method in this paper.

References

1. Li, W., Zhu, W., Wang, X., et al.: Text2DT: decision rule extraction technology for clinical medical text. J. Med. Inform. **43**(12), 16–22 (2022)

2. Zhu, W., Li, W., Wang, X., et al.: Extracting decision trees from medical texts: an overview of the Text2DT track in CHIP 2022. In: Health Information Processing: 8th China Conference, CHIP 2022, Hangzhou, China, October 21–23, 2022, Revised Selected Papers. Singapore: Springer Nature Singapore (2022)
3. Lu, Y., Liu, Q, Dai, D., et al.: Unified structure generation for universal information extraction. In: Proceedings of the 60th Annual Meeting of the Association for Computational Linguistics (Volume 1: Long Papers) (2022)
4. Zong, H., Lei, J., Li, Z, et al.: Overview of technology evaluation dataset for medical multimodal information extraction. J. Med. Inform. **43**(12), 2–5+22 (2022)

Research on Decision Tree Method of Medical Text Based on Information Extraction

Zihong Wu(✉)

1M Data Technology Co., Ltd., Beijing, China
wzh_home@163.com

Abstract. Extracting diagnosis and treatment decision trees from medical texts is a very meaningful thing. Recently, research in this area has just started. The general direction is to use pipeline extraction methods, which can be divided into two steps: triplet extraction and decision tree generation. However, in the previous research method, there are some problems in triplet extraction and decision tree generation, which lead to poor effect of the whole decision extraction. This paper improves in the following three directions: (1) adopts the pre-training method on the medical data set; (2) uses named entity recognition and biaffine to judge the relationship between entities in terms of triplet extraction; (3) adopts the pattern method to make the triples generate a decision tree. Through the above three improvements, it has achieved excellent performance on the 2022CHIP evaluation three data sets (Text2MDT) The medical pre-training model allows the model to have a deeper understanding of medical vocabulary and the dependencies between vocabulary; The triplet ex-traction method uses biaffine to judge that the entity relationship is suitable for the triplet extraction of the evaluation data set; The method using the pattern triplet is more expressive.

Keywords: triplet extraction · pretrain · decision tree

1 Instruction

Medical literature decision tree extraction is a meaningful topic of medical literature information extraction. It can help us learn medical knowledge and assist agent query through natural language processing. With the development of CDSS, medical text decision tree extraction also appeared. As early as 2009, Demner-Fushman D used natural language processing technology to help use text information to drive CDSS, focusing on the application of nlp technology (such as: text preprocessing, named entity recognition, context extraction, relationship extraction) to text information extraction, to extract relevant knowledge and apply it to the CDSS system, focusing on the logical process of front and back information, and the prototype of the text decision tree [1]. In 2013, Deleger L further standardized the extraction of medical text information, and

Supported by organization 1M Data Technology Co., Ltd.

B. Tang et al. (Eds.): CHIP 2022, CCIS 1773, pp. 127–133, 2023.
https://doi.org/10.1007/978-981-99-4826-0_12

measured the performance of medical text information extraction by evaluating a large number of natural language processing results, collecting medical records from the largest children's hospital in the United States, with about 5 million files, through Com-pared with the large-scale information extraction results of nlp and human processing, it is found that the effect is not much different, which makes the application of nlp in medical text information extraction more reliable [2]. In 2022, Li Wenfeng proposed to extract decision trees from medical texts and apply them to CDSS, thereby reducing the dependence of CDSS on experts for medical decision-making, and gave relevant data sets, evaluation indicators and methods [3–5]. In order to improve the performance of the model in the 2022CHIP evaluation 3, this paper makes the following improvements: (1) Adopt the pre-training method on the medical dataset; (2) In terms of triplet extraction, use named entity recognition and biaffine to judge the relationship between entities; (3) Use the pattern method to make the triples generate a decision tree. Text information extraction diagnosis and treatment decision tree can be divided into two sub-tasks: triplet extraction and decision tree construction. A series of triples are obtained by triplet extraction and aggregated into nodes, and then the connection between nodes is explored to form a diagnosis and treatment decision tree.

1.1 Triple Extraction

The basic granularity of a diagnosis and treatment decision tree is a triplet, and the accuracy of the triplet directly affects downstream tasks. The composition of triples is (entity, relation, entity). An entity is a meaningful segment that needs to be extracted directly from the text. Entities and relationships between entities are just two states in this paper, relationship exists, and relationship does not exist. A more conventional approach is to perform named entity recognition on the text first, and then judge whether the relationship between the two entities exists and extract them into triples if they exist. Due to the separation of named entity recognition and relationship discrimination between entities, it will cause errors in named entity recognition to be passed to relationship discrimination, so we usually put named entity recognition and relationship discrimination in the same model. For the study of dependency relationships, as early as 2017, Timothy Dozat used the biaffine model to construct syntactic relationships during dependency syntax analysis, and achieved the sota [6]. In 2019, Li Ying used the bert pre-training model instead of bilstm for text context semantic representation, which is very helpful for biaffine to capture lexical dependency information, which improves the effect of syntactic analysis [7] juntao yu in 2020, used the biaffine model for named entity recognition, modeled the internal dependencies of entities, and solved nesting problems [8]. In summary, the biaffine model can convert the sequence into a matrix, and then model the internal and external dependencies of the sequence. This article uses the biaffine model to model between entities (outside entity). At the same time, use medical text data to pre-train again on the basis of Roformerv2 pre-training model [9], so that it can be helpful for biaffine downstream tasks

1.2 Decision Tree Composition

After completing the steps of triplet extraction, the next step is to aggregate the discrete triplets into tree nodes, and calculate the cosine distance between the triplets, and merge them when the cosine distance reaches a certain threshold. When mining the relationship between nodes, let the nodes establish connections to form a graph. As long as the graph is reasonably defined, a decision tree can be obtained. The root node has no parent node, and the leaf node has no children. When decoding, the root node is decoded first, and then a tree is constructed according to the depth-first search algorithm until the leaf node is encountered.

2 Method

2.1 Medical Language Model Pre-training

In this paper, Roformerv2 is used as the initialization parameter of the pre-training model, and pre-training is performed on the medical dataset. The difference between medical data and general data is that medical data is more specialized. Modeling on medical data sets is more conducive to the model's understanding of professional knowledge in the medical field. In order to help the model understand the basic ability of medical language, this paper adopts the following methods, (1) mask token method, which is consistent with Bert's mask strategy, and maintains the model's ability to understand the vocabulary through sentence semantics, (2) text infilling method, using Poor Loose distribution mask a continuous token, let the model learn the length to be predicted, (3) divide the sentence into upper and lower sentences, mask part of the nouns in the previous sentence, and generate the next sentence.

2.2 Triple Extraction Method

The medical text sequence can capture the semantic information between the sequences through the pre-training model. As long as the objective function is reasonably designed for the downstream tasks, the model can play a very good role. Triple extraction is mainly to extract fragments and the association between fragments. A piece of text with a length of n has n(n+1) fragment combinations, and there are n(n+1)/2 combinations regardless of the direction factor. We only need to model meaningful fragment boundaries and relationships to complete our Target. Entity extraction involves the boundaries of entities in the text and the categories of entities, which can be divided into multi-task learning when modeling. Each task shares pre-trained model parameters, and subtasks have their own independent parameter space. In terms of multi-task sharing parameters, a text sequence obtains the representation of each token through the pre-training model. Entity boundary extraction task, each token is mapped by two dense maps to obtain the mapping H and T of the entity head and tail respectively, HUT is mapped to n*n*k intersection matrix, k = 2 represents whether the head and tail intersect, the intersection matrix has Symmetry, take the upper triangle and connect the cross-entropy loss function. Entity category discrimination task, take H and T splicing and pass through dense+softmax, then cross entropy. For the task of relation-ship between entities and entities, the tokens of the two entities are respectively taken through the biaffine model, and then it is judged whether the two entities are related. Specifically, as shown in Fig. 1

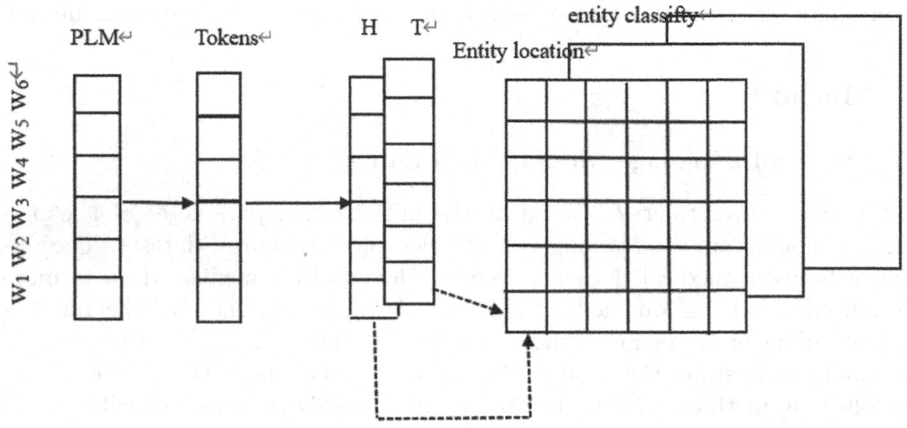

Fig. 1. Triple extraction is divided into three parts, entity location, entity classification, entity relationship reasoning

2.3 Pattern Triplets About the Method of Decision Tree Mining

Decision tree mining can be carried out after the triples are obtained. The common method is to take the last entity in the triples to represent the triples and text splicing, and take <s> and <e> to split the triples. When using this method, the last entity is not representative of a triplet. If the last entity of different triplets is the same, the above method will fail at this time. If the triplets are put together and there is no good way to connect them, the solution It is to use special tokens to connect triplets, and then learn these special tokens through the model, so that they have special meanings. Afterwards, the maximum pooling of the triplets is used to form a vector, and let it represent the triplets and put them into the bi-affine to judge the relationship between nodes.

3 Experiment

This article is mainly for the research on the three data sets of CHIP2022 evaluation, which is mainly divided into the improvement of triplet extraction and decision tree generation, so the experiment is divided into two parts. The amount of data is 300 training sets, 100 test sets, and 100 verification sets

3.1 About Triplet Experiment Evaluation, Experiment Comparison, and Result Analysis

The triplet experimental evaluation is measured by precision, recall, and F1 indicators. The experimental comparison with the current state-of-the-art relationship extraction UniRE [10] and TPLinker [11] models in the evaluation of the three data sets is shown in the following Table 1:

Table 1. the performance of different models in evaluating the relationship extraction

Model	precision	recall	F1
TPLinker	0.86719	0.86991	0.87072
UniRE	0.86349	0.85266	0.85804
CasDE	0.86271	0.86677	0.86474
This method	0.88329	0.89276	0.89807

Result analysis: In the three data sets of CHIP evaluation, the triplet elements are relatively single, such as (patient, clinical manifestation), (patient, treatment plan), (therapeutic drug, usage and dosage), (patient, therapeutic drug), (patient, prohibited drug). The patient only appears once in the text sequence. Faced with such a problem, the accuracy of named entity recognition is very high, The relationship between entities is also relatively simple, there are no multiple relationships, and the relationship between entities can be extracted by label combination is also relatively effective, It's just that there are two pairs of therapeutic drugs and their usage and dosage can't be aligned. You only need to judge whether there is a dependency relation-ship between the entity and the entity, and use the scheme in this paper to obtain better results.

3.2 Experimental Evaluation, Experimental Comparison, and Result Analysis of Decision Tree Generation

The evaluation indicators used in decision tree generation include node F1, diagnosis and treatment decision tree F1 (DTF1), decision path F1(DPF1), and decision tree edit distance (DTED). This experiment is mainly compared with the methods in Text2DT, such as seq2seq [12], seq2tree [13], text2dt. This experiment is detailed in Table 2.

Result analysis: This paper makes model improvements based on the characteristics of the three data sets of the 2022CHIP evaluation, so the performance is better than the Text2DT model. Seq2seq and seq2tree, because the current decoding result in the decoding stage will depend on the previous result, the previous result error is easy to pass backward. When Text2dt uses triples to generate pg decision tree, the last element in the triples is used to represent the triples.

Table 2. The performance of different models to generate decision trees

Model	Node F1	DTF1	DPF1	DTED
Seq2seq	0.6239	0.2700	0.4209	6.78
Seq2tree	0.6243	0.2700	0.4221	6.72
Text2dt	0.6763	0.3400	0.4658	5.74
This method	0.7399	0.3700	0.5271	5.41

The expressive ability is not strong, so the effect is not as good as this method. Moreover, this article uses medical data for pre-training. When the training set data is not much, pre-training can increase the model's understanding of the language and semantics of medical data, which is helpful for downstream tasks. Triple extraction is also modeled according to the characteristics of the data set, the effect is better than other models, and the text2dt triplet is not strong enough to express when generating a decision tree.

4 Conclusions

The improvement of the Text2DT method in this paper is superior to Text2DT in the performance of the three data sets of the 2022CHIP evaluation. Use medical datasets to pre-train the pre-trained model again, so that the model can have a deeper understanding of medical vocabulary and the dependencies between vocabulary; The triplet extraction method is improved to make it more suitable for the triplet extraction of the evaluation data set; Use the pattern triplet to generate a decision tree to make the triplet more expressive.
There are also deficiencies in this paper. This paper adopts pipeline modeling, and the triplet extraction task is separated from the diagnostic decision tree generation task, so that the triplet extraction error will be passed to the diagnostic decision tree generation task. In the future, the triplet Integration of extraction and diagnosis and treatment decision tree generation

References

1. Demner-Fushman, D., Chapman, W.W., McDonald, C.J.: What can natural language processing do for clinical decision support? J. Biomed. Inform **42**(5), 760–772. Epub 2009 Aug 13. PMID: 19683066; PMCID: PMC2757540. https://doi.org/10.1016/j.jbi.2009.08.007
2. Deleger, L., et al.: Large-scale evaluation of automated clinical note de-identification and its impact on information extraction. J. Am. Med. Inform. Assoc. **20**(1), 84–94. Epub 2012 August 2. PMID: 22859645; PMCID: PMC3555323 https://doi.org/10.1136/amiajnl-2012-001012
3. Zong, H, Lei, J, Li, Z, et al. Overview of technology evaluation dataset for medical multimodal information extraction. J. Med. Inform. **43**(12), 2–5+22 (2022)

4. Li, W., Zhu, W., Wang, X., et al.: Text2DT: decision rule extraction technology for clinical medical text .J. Med. Inform. **43**(12), 16–22 (2022)
5. Zhu, W., Li, W., Wang, X., et al.: Extracting decision trees from medical texts: an overview of the Text2DT track in CHIP 2022. In: Health Information Processing: 8th China Conference, CHIP 2022, Hangzhou, China, October 21–23, 2022, Revised Selected Papers. Singapore: Springer Nature Singapore (2022)
6. Dozat, T., Manning, C.: Deep biaffine attention for neural dependency parsing. In Proceedings of ICLR, 2017
7. Li, Y., Li, Z., Zhang, M., Wang, R., Li, S., Si, L.: Self-attentive Bi-affine dependency parsing. In: Proceedings of ICLR, 2019
8. Yu, J., Bohnet, B., Poesio, M.: Named entity recognition as dependency parsing. In: Proceedings of the 58th Annual Meeting of the Association for Computational Linguistics, pp. 6470–6476, Online. Association for Computational Linguistics (2020)
9. Su, J., Lu, Y., Pan, S., Wen, B., Liu, Y.: Roformerv2: a faster and better roformer. Technical report(2022)
10. Teo, T.W., Choy, B.H.: in. In: Tan, O.S., Low, E.L., Tay, E.G., Yan, Y.K. (eds.) Singapore Math and Science Education Innovation. ETLPPSIP, vol. 1, pp. 43–59. Springer, Singapore (2021). https://doi.org/10.1007/978-981-16-1357-9_3
11. 9. Wang, Y., Yu, B., Zhang, Y., Liu, T., Zhu, H., Sun, L.: TPLinker: single-stage joint extraction of entities and relations through token pair linking. In: Proceedings of the 28th International Conference on Computational Linguistics, pp. 1572–1582, Barcelona, Spain (Online). International Committee on Computational Linguistics (2020)
12. 10. Lei, W., Yan, W., Deng, C., et al.: Translating a math word problem to an expression Tree. In: Proceedings of the 2018 Conference on Empirical Methods in Natural Language Processing, Brussels: Association for Computational Linguistics, pp. 1064–1069 (2018)
13. 11. Xie, Z., Sun, S.: A goal-driven tree-structured neural model for math word problems. In: Proceedings of the Twenty-Eighth International Joint Conference on Artificial Intelligence. Macao: IJCAI, pp. 5299–5305 (2019)

OCR of Electronic Medical Document

Information Extraction of Medical Materials: An Overview of the Track of Medical Materials MedOCR

Lifeng Liu[1], Dejie Chang[1(✉)], Xiaolong Zhao[1], Longjie Guo[1], Mosha Chen[2], and Buzhou Tang[3]

[1] Beijing Universal Medical Assistance, Beijing 100020, China
changdejie2007@126.com
[2] Ali Yun Tianchi, Hangzhou 310000, China
[3] Pengcheng Laboratory, Harbin Institute of Technology, Shenzhen 518055, China

Abstract. In the medical and insurance industry, electronic medical record materials contain a lot of information, which can be extracted and applied to various businesses through artificial intelligence technology, which will greatly reduce labor costs and improve efficiency. However, it is difficult to extract. At present, most of them rely on manual input. Using Optical Character Recognition (OCR) and Natural Language Processing (NLP) technology to electronize and structure the information on these paper materials has gradually become a hot spot in the current industry. Based on this, we constructed a medical material information extraction data set Medical OCR dataset (MedOCR) [1], and we also held the "Medical inventory invoice OCR element extraction Task" evaluation competition based on the eighth China Health Information processing Conference (CHIP2022), in order to promote the development of medical material information extraction technology. A total of 18 teams participated in the competition, most of which used an OCR-based extraction system. For the evaluation index Acc, the best performing teams reached 0.9330 and 0.9076. The task of the competition focuses on information extraction technology, and MedOCR will be open for researchers to carry out related technical research for a long time.

Keywords: Artificial intelligence technology · Natural Language Processing · Optical Character Recognition · information extraction

1 Introduction

1.1 Background

At present, the medical records used in hospitals are still paper-based, in which the information includes: customer information, diagnostic information, medication information, cost information and so on. In the medical industry and insurance industry, this information has high commercial and scientific research value, and it is difficult to extract. At present, it still depends on manual input. With the gradual development and popularization of artificial intelligence technology such as OCR and NLP in production and

B. Tang et al. (Eds.): CHIP 2022, CCIS 1773, pp. 137–142, 2023.
https://doi.org/10.1007/978-981-99-4826-0_13

life, compared with the traditional manual input, the application of OCR and NLP technology can effectively improve work efficiency and reduce the training cost of business personnel. Using OCR and NLP technology to electronize and structure the information on these paper materials has gradually become a hot spot in the current industry.

MedOCR [1] provides four types of medical records: outpatient invoice, hospitalization invoice, drug purchase tax bill and discharge summary. The main purpose of this paper is to extract the fixed fields of these four types of materials and generate structured data, which has been explained in detail in the "Medical inventory invoice OCR element extraction Task" evaluation competition.

1.2 Objective

In cooperation with Ali Yun Tianchi, we jointly held the "Medical inventory invoice OCR element extraction Task" evaluation competition, which aims to promote the development of medical material information extraction technology. In this article, we will first give an overview of the tasks of MedOCR and how we prepare the data. Then we describe the number of teams participating in the competition and the methods of the teams with better performance, and finally we introduce the results.

2 Method

2.1 Task Overview

MedOCR provides out-patient invoices, hospitalization invoices, drug purchase tax tickets and discharge summary. The real pictures and labeled data of these four types of medical records are shared with all participating teams as training data sets. The participating teams use their own methods to extract the fixed fields and generate the final formatted data, and then calculate the accuracy of the generated formatted data and labeled data. Finally, the accuracy is used as the evaluation index to rank the team.

2.2 Data Preparation

The original data set of MedOCR comes from the Internet, with a total of 1700 pictures of four kinds of medical records, including discharge summary, drug purchase invoice, outpatient invoice and hospitalization invoice. Then we select fixed fields for each type of material to label. Finally, we divide the data set into three parts: training set, evaluation A list and evaluation B list. The training set is shared with the participating teams to learn. Evaluation A list is the comparison and verification of the methods used by the participating teams, and the evaluation B list is the final check of the methods used by the participating teams. The data distribution is shown in Table 1.

2.3 Baseline Method

We use the two-stage algorithm of Differentiable Binarization [2] for text detection and CRNN [3] for text recognition to realize OCR. Because of the extraction difficulties caused by irregular images, we use Bert [4] for text classification and LSTM-CRF [5] for named entity recognition to deal with the text extracted by OCR. The final accuracy is shown in Table 2.

Table 1. MedOCR data distribution table

Dataset name	Grading	Material category	Category quantity
Medical labeling task data set	Training set	Summary of discharge from hospital	200
		Drug purchase invoice	200
		Outpatient invoice	200
		Hospitalization invoice	400
	Evaluate list A	Summary of discharge from hospital	40
		Drug purchase invoice	40
		Outpatient invoice	40
		Hospitalization invoice	80
	Evaluate list B	Summary of discharge from hospital	100
		Drug purchase invoice	100
		Outpatient invoice	100
		Hospitalization invoice	200

Table 2. Effect of baseline

Material type	Accuracy
Summary of discharge from hospital	0.884
Drug purchase invoice	0.861
Outpatient invoice	0.793
Hospitalization invoice	0.920
Total	0.883

2.4 Evaluation Indicators

Accuracy can directly show the effect of the method of the participating team, so the accuracy is used as the evaluation index. For example, if the number of correct fields predicted is correct and the number of wrong fields predicted is error, the accuracy rate is the proportion of the number of correct fields predicted to the sum of the number of predicted correct fields and the number of predicted wrong fields. When both predicted values and correct values are "none", this value will not be included in the calculation. When the predicted value is completely consistent with the correct value, the prediction is judged to be correct, otherwise it is judged to be wrong.

3 Results and Discussion

3.1 Participating Teams

A total of 18 teams participated in this competition, and as there was no limit on the number of submissions, only the submission date was limited, so only the highest score submitted by the team was selected as the final score of the team, and 17 teams submitted valid results.

3.2 Team Performance and Ranking

As the scores of the teams at the bottom of the rankings are not ideal, we only show the names and results of the top 10 teams. Table 3 shows the evaluation of the final results of the A-list teams. Table 4 shows the evaluation of the final results of the teams on the B list.

Table 3. Evaluation of list A ranking

Rank	Team	Techniques	Acc
1	TBJK	OCR	0.9032
2	St	OCR	0.9003
3	tiny_piggy	Bert	0.8395
4	try_ocr	OCR	0.8332
5	BJTU	OCR	0.8265
6	INFINITY SECURITY	ISDONE	0.5902
7	安全部	E2E	0.5413
8	zut-2022-cv	OCR	0.4655
9	山东师范大学	MyOCR	0.4125
10	试一试	Bert	0.3394

3.3 System Descriptions

Since most teams have low scores, only two teams have scored more than baseline, and only one team has agreed to share the methods they use, so here are some ideas and methods for the first team.

ANTINS team

For the task of this competition, we provide two schemes to solve the problem, one is to use the scheme without OCR, OCR-Free Document Understanding Transformer [6], to map the image of the training set to embedding as the input of the encoder, and train the

Table 4. Evaluation of list B ranking

Rank	Team	Techniques	Acc
1	ANTINS	Bert	0.9330
2	太保科技	OCR	0.9076
3	试一试	OCR	0.6409
4	INFINITY SECURITY	ISDONE	0.6202
5	BJTU	OCR	0.5600
6	安全部	OCR	0.5074
7	zut-2022-cv	OCR	0.4705
8	山东师范大学	MyOCR	0.4530
9	test	OCR	0.3972
10	MVVM	OCR	0.3672

field marked token of the training set as the output of the decoder to get the final model. This scheme achieves good performance in speed and accuracy.

The other is a knowledge-based multi-modal, multi-architecture medical voucher element extraction solution, Exploiting Match Relevancy between Entities for Visual Information Extraction [7], which combines the multi-architecture capabilities of NLP and CV, using a super pre-trained entity extraction model and a multi-modal information extraction model. And the knowledge is injected and the master code is constructed, which can realize the knowledge-based model fusion controllably.

3.4 Evaluation Results

In the task of extracting OCR elements from medical inventory invoices, we found that most of the teams performed poorly, and the top two teams performed well, of which only one team was willing to share their plans and provided different ideas to solve the problem. The first scheme based on multi-mode is more accurate, but the amount of computation is larger, and the second is that the OCR-free scheme is faster and has less computation. The accuracy is not as high as that of the multimodal scheme in short, the two schemes have their own advantages and disadvantages.

4 Conclusions

This overview document summarizes the data collection and team participation tracking of medical materials MedOCR. It consists of 1700 medical record pictures of real scenes as the original data set, which contains a lot of complex and uncertain components, so it is difficult to extract information. Overall, 2 of the 18 teams were better than the baseline approach, and the top team offered two solutions. In view of the complexity of medical material photos, the MedOCR task is still challenging. The MedOCR task can continue to serve as a venue for researchers in the medical informatics community to develop and improve medical information extraction technologies.

Conflicts of Interest. None declared.

References

1. Zong, H., Lei, J., Li, Z., et al.: Overview of technology evaluation dataset for medical multimodal information extraction. J. Med. Indformatics **43**(12), 2–5+22 (2022)
2. Liu, L., Chang, D., Zhao, X., et al.: MedOCR: the dataset for extraction of optical character recognition elements for medical materials. J. Med. Indformatics **43**(12), 28–31 (2022)
3. Liao, M., Wan, Z., Yao, C., Chen, K., Bai, X.: Real-time scene text detection with differentiable binarization. In: AAAI 2020, pp. 11474–11481 (2020). https://ojs.aaai.org/index.php/AAAI/article/view/6812
4. Shi, B., Bai, X., Yao, C.: An end-to-end trainable neural network for image-based sequence recognition and its application to scene text recognition. IEEE Trans. Pattern Anal. Mach. Intell. **39**(11), 2298–2304 (2017). https://doi.org/10.1109/TPAMI.2016.2646371
5. Devlin, J., Chang, M.W., Lee, K., et al.: Bert: pre-training of deep bidirectional transformers for language understanding. NAACL-HLT (1) 4171–4186 (2019). https://doi.org/10.18653/v1/n19-1423
6. Huang, Z., Xu, W., Yu, K.: Bidirectional LSTM-CRF models for sequence tagging. CoRR abs/1508.01991 (2015). http://arxiv.org/abs/1508.01991
7. Kim, G., et al.: OCR-free document understanding transformer. https://arxiv.org/abs/2111.15664
8. Tang, G., et al.: MatchVIE: exploiting match relevancy between entities for visual information extraction. IJCAI 2021: 1039–1045. https://arxiv.org/abs/2106.12940

TripleMIE: Multi-modal and Multi Architecture Information Extraction

Boqian Xia, Shihan Ma, Yadong Li, Wenkang Huang, Qiuhui Shi, Zuming Huang, Lele Xie, and Hongbin Wang(✉)

AntGroup, Shanghai 200001, China
{xiaboqian.xbq,mashihan.msh,hongbin.whb}@antgroup.com

Abstract. The continuous development of deep learning technology makes it widely used in various fields. In the medical scene, electronic voucher recognition is a very challenging task. Compared with traditional manual entry, the application of OCR and NLP technology can effectively improve work efficiency and reduce the training cost of business personnel. Using OCR and NLP technology to digitize and structure the information on these paper materials has gradually become a hot spot in the current industry.

Evaluation task 4 (OCR identification of electronic medical paper documents (ePaper)) of CHIP2022 [15,16,25] requires extracte 87 fields from the four types of medical voucher materials, including discharge summary, outpatient invoice, drug purchase invoice, and inpatient invoice. This task is very challenging because of the various types of materials, noise-contained data, and many categories of target fields.

To achieve the above goals, we propose a knowledge-based multi-modal and multi-architecture medical voucher information extraction method, namely TripleMIE, which includes I2SM: Image to sequence model, L-SPN: Large scale PLM-based span prediction net, MMIE: multi-modal information extraction model, etc. At the same time, a knowledge-based model integration module named KME is proposed to effectively integrate prior knowledge such as competition rules and material types with the model results. With the help of the above modules, we have achieved excellent results on the online official test data, which verifies the performance of the proposed method.(https://tianchi.aliyun.com/dataset/131815#4)

Keywords: CHIP 2022 · OCR identification · TripleMIE

1 Introduction

The electronic medical voucher recognition takes the photos or scanned photos of the voucher as the input, and requires extraction of the specified fields from the above data sources, such as gender, age, hospital name, bill number, payee, and other fields. Electronic structured data is generated by electronic medical

B. Xia and S. Ma–Contribute equally to this work.

B. Tang et al. (Eds.): CHIP 2022, CCIS 1773, pp. 143–153, 2023.
https://doi.org/10.1007/978-981-99-4826-0_14

voucher recognition. At present, when dealing with electronic bills and medical materials, most researchers first perform OCR identification on the materials to identify the corresponding text [21] and then use some entity extraction methods to extract the fields contained in the materials as entities. At the same time, some researchers proposed multi-modal models to improve performance [7].

Electronic medical voucher recognition is a very challenging task [2,17], which has the following difficulties: the discrete data of life insurance electronic medical voucher lacks national standards, the format and fields of each region are different, and the format of information contained is also quite different; Secondly, the resolution and shooting angle of the electronic medical voucher photos are different, and the image quality is also different, which poses a new challenge to recognition. In addition, some materials may contain a certain tilt angle, which brings trouble to subsequent recognition; In terms of data, due to the limited number of materials in each format, the long tail phenomenon of data is relatively serious; Finally, the annotation data of this task contains limited information [5,6]. For a material, its annotation data only includes its corresponding fields and values and does not include the location of this information corresponding to the original material.

To deal with the above problems, we proposed a multi-modal and multi-architecture information extraction model. First, we introduce an end-to-end extraction model, which takes material images as input and uses a transformer encoder to get the encoding information of the pictures. Then, we input the encoding information into the encoder and guide the model to generate corresponding fields through different prompt information. We call it the OCR-free model [9]; As we all know, the corresponding text in the picture also contains rich information. To make better use of it, we also introduced the OCR-based extraction module. Specifically, we used the OCR model to obtain the text contained in the materials. With the use of the grid-based OCR re-ordering method, we perform a checking and correction process of the raw OCR results. The corrected OCR results are then input into two models, namely a large-scale PLM-based span prediction network and a multi-modal information extraction model. Finally, we creatively propose the Knowledge-based model ensemble architecture, which integrates the results of the above multiple models on the premise of combining the competition rules and business prior knowledge.

In the end, the proposed model has achieved good results in both the leaderboard phase A and the leaderboard phase B. At the same time, we also proved the contribution of each module in our framework to the final test results through detailed ablation experiments.

2 Related Works

2.1 Optical Character Recognition

Optical Character Recognition (OCR) converts images of handwritten or printed text into text that can be encoded by a machine. This technology can be applied to text recognition of scanned documents and pictures. Generally, optical character recognition consists of two parts: text detection and text recognition. For text detection, the detector locates the specific position of the text segment in the image, and the granularity can be the text line level or the word level. Most current solutions treat this task as an object detection problem with specific optimizations for text problems. PSENet [22] proposed the post-processing of progressive scale expansion for improving detection accuracy. Specifically, PSENet [22] used the progressive scale expansion method by segmenting the text instances with different scale kernels. This method used new post-processing algorithms for the segmentation results, resulting in lower inference speed. Instead, DBnet [12] focuses on improving the segmentation results by including the binarization process in the training period, without the loss of the inference speed. In particular, even with a lightweight backbone (ResNet-18), DBnet [12] can achieve competitive performance on the testing datasets with real-time inference speed. Text recognition generally converts visual signals of text images into natural language symbols by a text recognizer. This task usually uses an encoder-decoder architecture. Most existing methods use a CNN-based encoder to encode an image into a feature space, and then apply an RNN-based decoder to extract characters from the features. Recently, to improve efficiency, many SOTA models have adopted the Transformer architecture. At the same time, they have begun to explore the use of self-supervised image pre-training methods for text recognition. For example, researchers at Microsoft Research Asia have conducted several studies focusing on text recognition tasks. They proposed the first end-to-end Transformer-based text recognition OCR model (TrOCR) [11] using the pre-trained method.

2.2 Visual Document Understanding

Recently, visual document understanding has attracted the attention of numerous researchers. The core of visual document understanding research is how to make full use of the multi-modal features of document images. The LayoutLM series models (LayoutLM v1-v3) [3,8,23] proposed by Microsoft are representative models for visual document understanding tasks. The LayoutLM series models have excellent performance and are widely used by industry and academia. These models use the output obtained through OCR technology and images together as the input, and then the ability is obtained to understand documents through a series of pre-training tasks. Finally, the models are finetuned on downstream tasks for the application. LayoutXLM [24] is the multilingual version of LayoutLMv2 [23]. This is a multi-modal pre-trained model for multilingual document understanding, which aims to bridge the language barriers for visually-rich document understanding. They achieved impressive results by successfully combining textual, layout, and visual features. However, The above models utilize the position embeddings to incorporate the sequence information, neglecting the noise of improper reading order obtained by OCR tools. Therefore, a robust layout-aware multi-modal network named XYLayoutLM [3]is proposed to capture and leverage rich layout information from proper reading orders produced by Augmented XYCut. The above methods follow a pipeline consisting of applying OCR followed by BERT-like transformers. The above-mentioned document understanding methods relying on OCR technology are complex and expensive. Some recent works have been proposed to simplify the complex document parsing process. The most representative of these is Donut [9], which is an end-to-end document understanding work. It is a new OCR-free visual document understanding model to address the problems induced by the OCR-dependency. The model is based on Transformer-only architecture, following the huge success in vision and language. Donut [9] model presented a minimal baseline including a simple architecture and pre-training method. Despite its simplicity, Donut [9] model shows comparable or better overall performance than previous methods.

3 The Proposed Method

3.1 Data Construction

Data preparation-related work consists of two parts: span prediction net related data processing and multi-modal related data preprocessing to enable the data provided by the sponsor to adapt to the input of the OCR-based model. In the annotation data provided by the sponsor, a picture corresponds to a series of key-value pairs stored in a CSV file with OCR recognition results of the pictures not provided, which also increases the difficulty of data processing. As a result, we need to perform OCR recognition first on all pictures to obtain all the corresponding text bounding boxes and recognition results, which together with the original picture and CSV recognition results serve as the information source for data processing.

Span Prediction Net Related Data Processing. Span prediction net is generally a named entity recognition task. In this task, we need to treat the value in all key-value pairs corresponding to the image as a span in the text. Here, we further simplify the problem and consider all the spans as continuous spans. For each span, we can regard the corresponding key as the type of the span. Specifically, we adopt a greedy matching strategy, combining the relative position of the span in the original text, and discarding the span whose relative position of context exceeds a certain position. However, some values cannot be searched in the OCR results due to some reasons, such as serious shooting tilt, blurred pictures, occlusion, and dislocation of OCR recognition results; In addition, the matching method cannot be used to label data for values that occur more than once, such as the default amount and some personal names. To solve the above problems, we first use greedy matching to label fields that appear only once. For the remaining fields, we use manual verification to fine-calibrate the data.

Data Preprocessing of Multi-modal Model. For multi-modal training data, we expect to collect a batch of medical-related texts from the open-source corpus in the form of labeled data, then use it to construct pseudo-labeled data to improve the generalization ability of the model [4,18]. Specifically, when constructing training data, we will mainly consider four variables, namely, layout information, material information, background information, and text information. We first randomly generate some layouts, then apply the layout to a certain material, combined it with the randomly generated background information, and finally draw the text on the picture according to the layout; In this way, we can construct a large number of labeled data and use them for training multi-modal models.

3.2 Large-scale PLM-based Span Prediction Net (L-SPN)

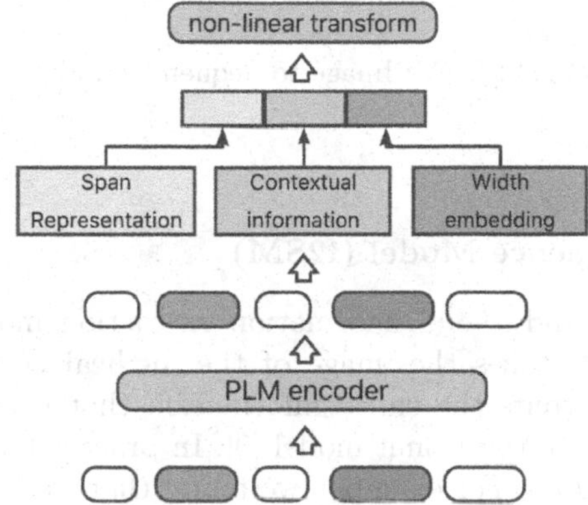

Fig. 1. L-SPN: Large-scale PLM based Span Prediction Net

The purpose of L-SPN is to input a sequence of tokens and output several consecutive pieces of text, each piece corresponding to a type of information, after being identified by the model [19]. For a medical voucher material, we first get the corresponding text recognition results through OCR recognition, then use the bounding box correction method [1], combined with prior knowledge, to rearrange the orders of each minimum unit text bounding box identified by OCR to get smoother full-text recognition results. Text T enters a transformer encoder after tokenization to get the embedding of each token. With a maximum span length set, we could get all continuous substrings that are less than the maximum length from the original text, each of which is a candidate span. For the model to learn the length information of the span, we innovatively introduced an additional embedding table: width embedding, through the width embedding we could obtain the embedding of the span length. The embedding is concatenated with the token embedding information of the candidate span to get the unified embedding of the span. Next, we use a non-linear classifier to determine whether the span is an entity and, if so, what type it corresponds to (Figs. 1 and 2).

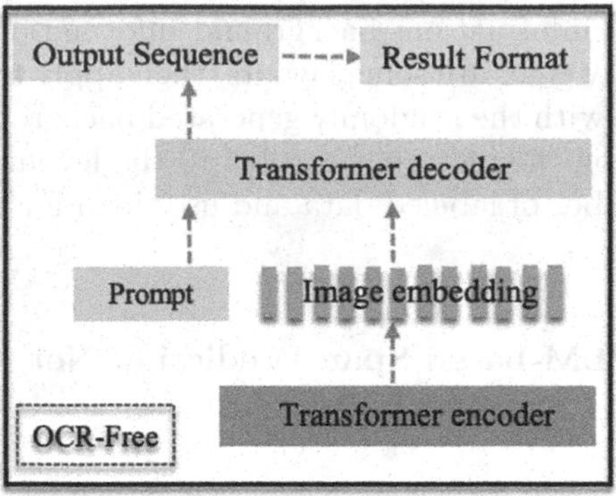

Fig. 2. I2SM: Image to Sequence Model

3.3 Image to Sequence Model (I2SM)

I2SM is a basic and end-to-end information extraction module in our overall solution. This module takes the image of the medical certificate material as input and directly outputs the entity information that needs to be extracted. This module is based on the Donut model [9]. In practical application, we have made some optimizations. For example, we found that the model is sensitive to the characteristics of the input image, so we added random data augmentation during training. In addition, we found that the vocabulary corresponding to the official pre-training model lacks a lot of words in the medical field. To solve this problem, we expanded the vocabulary of the model, which can greatly improve the information extraction accuracy of the model. At the same time, the training code is also optimized to increase the training speed and improve the efficiency of model training (Fig. 3).

3.4 Multi-modal Information Extraction Model (MMIE)

MMIE is a multi-modal information extraction module that depends on OCR. In this module, we refer to the MatchVIE [20] model and the LayoutLM series model [3,8,23]. It consists of a feature extraction backbone and two specific branches of relevancy evaluation and entity recognition, respectively. The feature extraction backbone network fully considers the multi-modal features of position, and image, as well as the correlation between them. Local and non-local features are captured by the backbone. Then the relevancy evaluation branch is based on a graph module to model the overall layout information of documents and obtain the key-value matching probability. Meanwhile, an entity recognition branch is used to solve the sequence labels of standalone text segments.

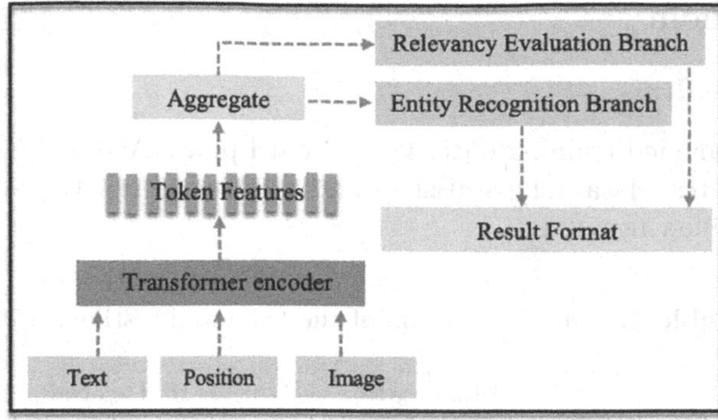

Fig. 3. MMIE: multi-modal Information Extraction Model

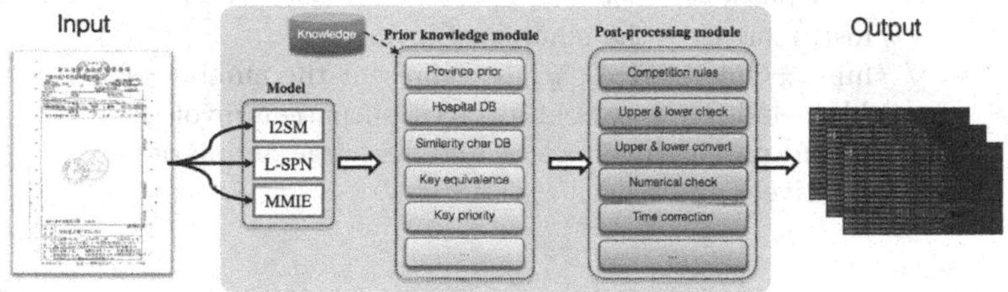

Fig. 4. KME: Knowledge-based Model Ensemble

3.5 Knowledeg-based Model Ensemble (KME)

A knowledge-based model integration module is proposed to make full use of the prior knowledge of medical voucher materials and achieve better model integration results. This module is equivalent to integrating multi-modal and multi-architecture information extraction modules and adding knowledge injection and post-processing modules. The KME module takes the images of voucher materials as input and directly outputs the result file in the specified format, as shown in Fig. 4. The prior knowledge module processes the prior knowledge of medical voucher materials obtained by data analysis into corresponding functions or databases. In the model ensemble, prior knowledge and the confidence of the model in specific fields are combined to make corresponding trade-offs. At the same time, the fields will be standardized by looking up tables to avoid the impact of text recognition errors. For example, we have built a database of hospital names and a database of similar words and easily mistaken words in the medical field. The post-processing module further improves the results of model recognition. First, we need to process the results of the algorithm model according to the format and rules specified in the competition. In addition, a series of post-processing rules are added to help improve the model results, such as uppercase and lowercase verification, uppercase and lowercase conversion, time correction, and value verification.

4 Experiment

4.1 Data Analysis

The sponsor provided training data, leaderboard phase A test data, and leaderboard phase B test data. The statistics and distribution of the above data are shown in the following table.

Table 1. Data distribution of the train and testing set.

Type	#Inst	#Inp	#Out	#Med	#Dis
Train	1000	14874	7004	2976	1600
Test phase A	200	2960	1360	320	320
Test phase B	500	7400	3400	800	800

#Inst. represents the number of instances.
#Inp., #Out., #Med., #Dis. represent the number of fields included in inpatient invoices, outpatient invoices, medicine purchasing invoices, and discharge summaries, respectively.

Analyzing the data, we can find that training (and test data) all contain four types of materials, and the number of fields to be extracted contained in each type of material is generally distributed evenly. In the training data, the number of inpatient invoice fields is about 9.29 times that of discharge summary fields.

4.2 Implementation Details

For L-SPN module, we encode the original text sequence T with a roberta-large-wwm [13] encoder, for all candidates sampled from T, we adopt a max pooling on the embedding of the first and last token of the span, represents as E_s, then concatenate it with the width embedding E_w:

$$E = \mathbf{concatanate}(E_s, E_w) \tag{1}$$

Then input E into a non-linear layer for multi-classification, and we can get whether the corresponding span is an entity and what its corresponding type is according to the classification results.

In the I2SM module, we refer to the Donut [9] model, use the Swin Transformer [14] as the visual encoder, and use BART [10] as the decoder. Then the model was trained on the training set for 200 epochs. In the MMIE module, we follow the LayoutLM series work [3,8,23], using BERT as the backbone of multi-modal information extraction, and adding the relevant head of entity recognition. In the OCR module, we use the PSENet [22] as the text detection model. Microsoft's TrOCR model [11] is used as the text recognition model. All the models are trained on the Chinese medical field certificate material dataset to obtain the best model performance.

4.3 Evaluation Metrics

The performance of the model on the test dataset is evaluated using accuracy. Accuracy is described as follows:

$$Accuracy = \frac{TruePositives}{TruePositives + FalsePositives} \tag{2}$$

It should be noted that if both the predicted value and the correct value are None, then this entity will not be included in the calculation result. If the predicted value is the same as the correct value, it is judged that the prediction of this entity is correct (Table 2).

4.4 Experiment Results

Table 2. ablation tests on the main components.

Settings	I2SM	LSPN	MMIE	KME	Accuracy
w/o I2SM	✗	✔	✔	✔	0.8559
w/o LSPN	✔	✗	✔	✔	0.7737
w/o MMIE	✔	✔	✗	✔	0.8046
w/o KME	✔	✔	✔	✗	0.7923
ALL	✔	✔	✔	✔	**0.9241**

In this section, we conducted ablation tests on the main components to study the impact of each specific component. In the experiment, only one component is removed at a time and other components remain unchanged. The specific results are shown in Table 1. As the results show, each component significantly impacts the final result. Algorithm models of different architectures will play different roles in different cases and fields. At the same time, the module based on prior knowledge and post-processing rules greatly improves the final results. The tests above prove our overall solution's effectiveness and complementarity of each module model.

5 Conclusion

This paper proposes a new method for extracting fields from electronic medical vouchers. We innovatively propose a multi-modal and multi-architecture extraction framework, which includes the end-to-end model of OCR-free, the span prediction model of OCR based, and the MMKV multi-modal extraction model. We use a model fusion method based on prior knowledge to fuse the results of multiple models with business knowledge and game rules. The above framework can effectively reduce the negative impact on the results due to inconsistent data standards, small sample size, shooting angle, style deviation, etc., and effectively improve the recognition effect of the model on various types of medical vouchers. Experimental results show that the proposed model can effectively extract structured information from electronic medical vouchers, and achieve high accuracy.

References

1. Chiron, G., Doucet, A., Coustaty, M., Moreux, J.P.: Icdar 2017 competition on post-ocr text correction. In: 2017 14th IAPR International Conference on Document Analysis and Recognition (ICDAR), vol. 1, pp. 1423–1428. IEEE (2017)
2. Ford, E., Carroll, J.A., Smith, H.E., Scott, D., Cassell, J.A.: Extracting information from the text of electronic medical records to improve case detection: a systematic review. J. Am. Med. Inf. Assoc. **23**(5), 1007–1015 (2016)
3. Gu, Z., et al.: Xylayoutlm: towards layout-aware multimodal networks for visually-rich document understanding. In: Proceedings of the IEEE/CVF Conference on Computer Vision and Pattern Recognition, pp. 4583–4592 (2022)
4. Guo, Z., Li, X., Huang, H., Guo, N., Li, Q.: Deep learning-based image segmentation on multimodal medical imaging. IEEE Trans. Radiat. Plasma Med. Sci. **3**(2), 162–169 (2019)
5. Gurulingappa, H., Mateen-Rajpu, A., Toldo, L.: Extraction of potential adverse drug events from medical case reports. J. Biomed. Semant. **3**(1), 1–10 (2012)
6. Hahn, U., Oleynik, M.: Medical information extraction in the age of deep learning. Yearbook Med. Inf. **29**(01), 208–220 (2020)
7. Hallett, C.: Multi-modal presentation of medical histories. In: Proceedings of the 13th International Conference on Intelligent user Interfaces, pp. 80–89 (2008)
8. Huang, Y., Lv, T., Cui, L., Lu, Y., Wei, F.: Layoutlmv3: pre-training for document AI with unified text and image masking. In: Proceedings of the 30th ACM International Conference on Multimedia (2022)
9. Kim, G., et al.: OCR-free document understanding transformer. In: Avidan, S., Brostow, G., Cissé, M., Farinella, G.M., Hassner, T. (eds.) Computer Vision - ECCV 2022. ECCV 2022. LNCS, vol. 13688, pp 498–517. Springer, Cham (2022). https://doi.org/10.1007/978-3-031-19815-1_29
10. Lewis, M., et al.: Bart: denoising sequence-to-sequence pre-training for natural language generation, translation, and comprehension. arXiv preprint arXiv:1910.13461 (2019)
11. Li, M., et al.: Trocr: transformer-based optical character recognition with pre-trained models. arXiv preprint arXiv:2109.10282 (2021)
12. Liao, M., Wan, Z., Yao, C., Chen, K., Bai, X.: Real-time scene text detection with differentiable binarization. In: Proceedings of the AAAI Conference on Artificial Intelligence, vol. 34, pp. 11474–11481 (2020)
13. Liu, Y., et al.: Roberta: A robustly optimized bert pretraining approach (2019)
14. Liu, Z., et al.: Swin transformer: Hierarchical vision transformer using shifted windows. In: Proceedings of the IEEE/CVF International Conference on Computer Vision, pp. 10012–10022 (2021)
15. Liu, L., Chang, D., Z.X.E.A.: Information extraction of medical materials: an overview of the track of medical materials medocr. In: Health Information Processing: 8th China Conference, CHIP 2022, Hangzhou, China, Revised Selected Papers. Springer Nature Singapore, Singapore, 21–23 October 2022

16. Liu, L., Chang, D., Z.X.e.a.: Medocr: the dataset for extraction of optical character recognition elements for medical materials. J. Med. Inf. **43**(12), 28–31 (2022)
17. Ruan, W., Appasani, N., Kim, K., Vincelli, J., Kim, H., Lee, W.S.: Pictorial visualization of EMR summary interface and medical information extraction of clinical notes. In: 2018 IEEE International Conference on Computational Intelligence and Virtual Environments for Measurement Systems and Applications (CIVEMSA), pp. 1–6. IEEE (2018)
18. Sharma, K., Giannakos, M.: Multimodal data capabilities for learning: what can multimodal data tell us about learning? Br. J. Educ. Technol. **51**(5), 1450–1484 (2020)
19. Tan, C., Qiu, W., Chen, M., Wang, R., Huang, F.: Boundary enhanced neural span classification for nested named entity recognition. In: Proceedings of the AAAI Conference on Artificial Intelligence, vol. 34, pp. 9016–9023 (2020)
20. Tang, G., et al.: Matchvie: exploiting match relevancy between entities for visual information extraction. arXiv preprint arXiv:2106.12940 (2021)
21. Thompson, P., McNaught, J., Ananiadou, S.: Customised ocr correction for historical medical text. In: 2015 Digital Heritage, vol. 1, pp. 35–42. IEEE (2015)
22. Wang, W., et al.: Shape robust text detection with progressive scale expansion network. In: Proceedings of the IEEE/CVF Conference on Computer Vision and Pattern Recognition, pp. 9336–9345 (2019)
23. Xu, Y., et al.: Layoutlmv2: multi-modal pre-training for visually-rich document understanding. arXiv preprint arXiv:2012.14740 (2020)
24. Xu, Y., et al.: Layoutxlm: multimodal pre-training for multilingual visually-rich document understanding. arXiv preprint arXiv:2104.08836 (2021)
25. Zong, H., Lei, J., L.Z.E.A.: Overview of technology evaluation dataset for medical multimodal information extraction. J. Med. Inf. **43**(12), 2–5+22 (2022)

Multimodal End-to-End Visual Document Parsing

Yujiang Lu[1](✉), Weifeng Qiu[1], Yinghua Hong[1], and Jiayi Wang[2]

[1] Infinity Security, Hangzhou, China
yujiang_lu@163.com
[2] Wenzhou Medical College, Wenzhou, China

Abstract. The record meterials used in some industries including medical service and insurance, whose information has high commercial and scientific research value, are still mainly paper-based. Recent progress in deep learning makes it easier to parse visually-rich document. Compared with traditional manual input, the application of this technology contributes to improvement of work efficiency and reduction of the training cost of business personnel. In previous work, the task of visual document parsing was divided into two stages which are composed of Optical Character Recognition (OCR) and Natural language understanding (NLU). In order to solve a series of problems in OCR, such as high computational costs, multi-language inflexibility and backward propagation of OCR errors, OCR-free multimodal visual document understanding method based on deep learning has been proposed recently. Through fine-tuning the pre-trained model, it can perform well in many downstream tasks. However, such approach is still limited in the specific context by 1) the language and context in which the encoder and decoder are pre-trained; 2) the image input size of the pre-trained encoder. In view of the above two problems, in this paper, we put forward the corresponding solutions, as a result, our proposed scheme won the second place in the "Identification of Electronic Medical Paper Documents (ePaper)" (IEMPD) task in the Eighth China Health Information Processing Conference (CHIP 2022) in an end-to-end way.

Keywords: Visual Document Parsing · Document Information Extraction · Optical Character Recognition · End-to-End

1 Introduction

With the rapid development of computers, more and more documents are stored, transmitted and used in the form of electronic version. However, documents in the modern production environments, such as outpatient medical records, inspection reports, receipts and invoices in the medical industry, still exist in large quantities in paper form and are commonly used. Whether it is electronic document images, screenshots or paper document photos, in order to extract useful and structured information, Visual Document Parsing (VDP) has become

B. Tang et al. (Eds.): CHIP 2022, CCIS 1773, pp. 154–163, 2023.
https://doi.org/10.1007/978-981-99-4826-0_15

an significant task for industry, and it is also a challenging topic for researchers. Information extraction [4,13] is one of the important applications of VDP.

In this work, our method is based on the model (Donut) architecture and trained weights provided in [7]. This paper details our various attempts and tuning schemes for the IEMPD task scenario in CHIP 2022 [10]. The work of this paper is summarized as follows:

- We build an offline document image generation tool, and use it to make a visual document dataset, VDDATA (VD), which includes 100,000 image-text pairs.
- By appropriately expanding the Chinese corpus and reducing the text size in pixels, we effectively solve the problem that the small word pixels could lead to misrecognition, fully take advantage of the representation ability of the model for small size character images, and greatly increase the training speed and inference speed of the model with almost no loss of performance.
- The experiment results on VD show that the proposed scheme enhances the performance of the model in the specific context of Chinese. The results on the IEMPD task show that the end-to-end model architecture we adopt can benefit well from the large model itself and large-scale pre-training, has a high upper bound and strong scalability.

2 Related Work

VDP methods are generally implemented in two ways: one-stage manner [7] and two-stage manner [3,4,6,14,15]. The traditional two-stage methods divide the VDP task into two steps: 1) reading the document image for texts; 2) parsing the visual document for holistic semantic information. They commonly rely on deep-learning-based OCR model [1,2] for the task of text reading and focus on modeling the semantic understanding part. One-stage methods are typically based on multi-modal models, which can omit the multi-classification process of OCR. They focus on modeling the visual semantic understanding of document images and the textual expression of visual words. Such one-stage methods effectively get rid of the limitations of OCR-based VDP model in computational cost, multi-language flexibility and propagation of errors in the previous stage.

But there are still limits to such a scheme. On the one hand, the pre-trained model is limited by the language scene during training. The fine-tuned model is required to have sufficient robust performance in specific language and context while retaining the benefits of large models and large-scale training. On the other hand, it is limited by the size of the document image input of the pre-trained model, the smaller image input can lead to the difficulty for the model to recognize characters, although such pixel size of the text is sufficient for general OCR models. The large size of the image input also leads to a great increase in the training and inference time of the model, which makes it difficult to be applied in industry.

3 Proposed Scheme

3.1 Data Generation

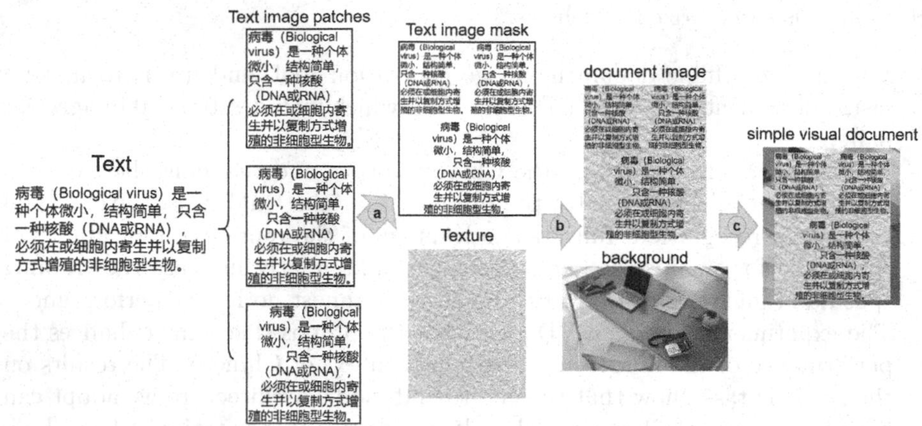

Fig. 1. Overview of our visual document generation method. Step (a) randomly reorganizes the text image patches with different alignments and fonts. Step (b) mixes the text image mask with texture image properly. Step (c) puts the document image into a natural background, we also randomly do some digital image transformations, light and shadow changes and so on, to make it as realistic as possible.

Synthesized document images should reflect realness of texts. There are related work of text image generator [16], but our main purpose is to expand the vocabulary of the model's tokenizer and make the model understand various Chinese word, so we try to avoid complex synthesis steps, and only implement the necessary parts by ourselves. The method of document image generation in this paper is shown in Fig. 1.

First, we need to convert the Chinese text collected from the wiki corpus into optical character images. We can easily control the appearance of the text image patch by configuring the number of characters in a line and basic character elements such as the size, spacing and font. We then simulate the creation of a document by simply arranging the text image patches randomly in rows or columns to recover the unique layout information of the "document". Second, we mix the generated binarized black-and-white text image with layout information with paper-like texture images in a random and reasonable ratio, which helps us generate document images without background. Finally, we put the document image into the background image with appropriate size and crop after the steps of projection transformation, perspective transformation and so on. In order to make the image more realistic, we add the effect of illumination shadow to it. We used a curve to divide the two regions of the image, and the curve obeying conventional curves such as linear, inverse, and exponential. From these two regions, we can generate a shadow mask. We make one region black and the other white, smooth them with a Gaussian blur, and blend them into the document image with the background, as a result, realistic visual documents with natural background are born.

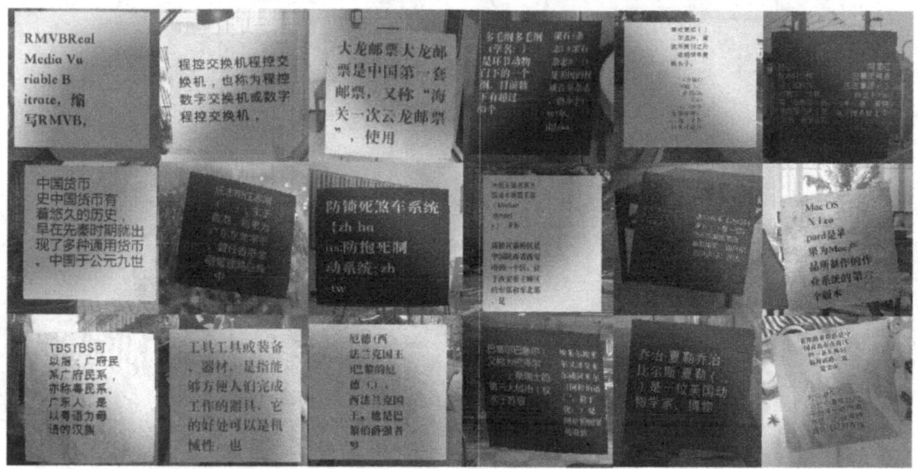
RMVBReal Media Va riable B itrate，缩 写RMVB，
程控交换机程控交 换机，也称为程控 数字交换机或数字 程控交换机，
大龙邮票大龙邮 票是中国第一套 邮票，又称“海 关一次云龙邮票 ”，使用
中国货币 史中国货币有 着悠久的历史， 早在先秦时期就出 现了多种通用货币 ，中国于公元九世
防锁死煞车系统
工具工具或装备 ，器材，是指能 够方便人们完成 工作的器具，它 的好处可以是机 械性，也

Fig. 2. Examples of the dataset VDDATA (VD).

In order to make the model achieve the goal of recognizing more characters, we use over 10 millon Chinese sentences, dozens of natural background pictrues and dozens of texture pictures to generate 100,000 document image data as shown in Fig. 2. The shape of these images is 224×224, and the smaller optical character size in the dataset is about 5×5, which is large enough for common OCR tasks.

3.2 Multimodal End-to-End Method

Referring to and basing on the work in [7], our method adopts encoder-decoder structure, as shown in Fig. 3, which visually encode the image and then send it to the language model decoder to generate the text. The generated text is the information extracted by the competition requirements, encoded in xml format and concatenated, like "<age>52</age><hospital_name>Affiliated hospital of Jilin University</hospital_name>$\cdots$".

Specifically, our approach is as follows. For every input image $I \in \mathbb{R}^{H \times W \times C}$, where H and W demote the resolutions and C denotes the channels of image, we first sequentially crop it into a sequence of image patches $P \in I^L_{patch}$, where L denotes the sentence length. For a sequence of image patches P, the backbone viewed as the encoder produces a sequence of visual feature words of size $F \in \mathbb{R}^{L \times C'}$, where C' denotes the channels of feature word. Our method then feeds

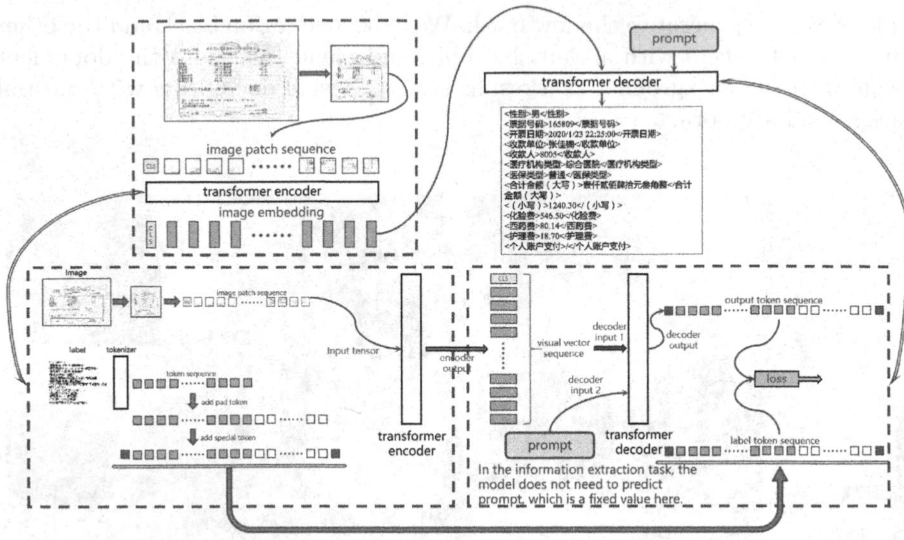

Fig. 3. Overview of our multimodal end-to-end method.

these visual feature words F into a language model for textual decoding. As a result, we get the output text $S \in \mathbb{L}^L$, where $\mathbb{L}$ denotes Chinese character set.

We take the same as the pre-training task as in the original work, so we load the trained weights from the original work into the model. However, since the weight is pre-trained in a multilingual environment, we decide to fine-tune the model with the generated dataset VD described in Sect. 3.1. The model is trained to read all the text in the image in the regular reading order (basically from top-left to bottom right). The objective is to minimize the cross-entropy loss of next text part by jointly conditioning on the image and previous contexts. This task can be interpreted as a pseudo-OCR task. The model is trained as a visual language model on a visual corpus, i.e., document images.

4 Experiment

For such an end-to-end model, there are many downstream tasks that can be done after it pre-training. For the question answering task (QA), we can prompt the model for training by setting prompt sequence. For classification task, we can pool the output of the encoder and then directly connect it to the classification head to complete the classification task. For the information extraction task, we can fix the prompt part and train the model to output the formatted text of the target. The model we used for the information extraction task is also benefiting from large-scale model pre-training.

Table 1. Basic information of datasets used in this work.

Dataset	Images (k)	Size	Storage usage (MB)
CHIP2022	1	480p-4k	645
VD	100	224*224	13160

4.1 Datasets

For the pseudo-OCR pre-training task, we adopt the dataset VD made by ourselves. VD consists of 100,000 document images with different Chinese texts, which are the same size 224 × 224. It contains over 10 million sentence, which ensures that the model can learn Chinese characters as widely as possible. It also makes the vocabulary of the tokenizer moderately expanded.

For the information extraction task, we only use 1000 training samples provided by CHIP 2022 organizers, which contain several kinds of medical documents [11,19]. There are 200 discharge summaries, 200 drug purchase tax invoices, 200 outpatient invoices, and 400 inpatient invoices in them. The data in this dataset is apparently augmented, where the same image material is used to make document images with different text content. Tabel 1 lists some basic information about the datasets we use in our scheme.

4.2 Settings

In order to make the framework more suitable for information extraction task, we use Swin Transformer [12] (Swin) as the visual encoder and use Bart [8] as the textual decoder, which both have been pre-trained based on pseudo-OCR task in work [7]. We have also tried some other backbones [9] and decoders, but none of them performed better than Swin and Bart. We think that this result is closely related to the large-scale pseudo-OCR pre-training task.

Table 2. Training settings of our proposed model.

Settings	Pseudo-OCR task	Information extraction task
Dataset	VD	CHIP 2022
Input size	224*224	1280*960
Batch size	128	4
Epoch	20	20
Optimizer	Adam	Adam
Loss function	cross-entropy	cross-entropy
Learning rate	3e–5	3e–5
Weight decay	1e–5	0
Warm-up steps	1500	300

As in Tabel 2, the training of both tasks consists of 20 epochs without early stopping. At the beginning of the first epoch, we set up some warm-up steps, and the number of warm-up steps depends on the total amount of data, the batch size and the number of epochs. We use adaptive moment estimation (Adam) as the optimizer and use cross-entropy loss as the loss function. We set $learning\ rate = 3e-5$, and learning rate first increases linearly to the preset value during the warm-up steps, then it decays as a cosine function. For pseudo-OCR task, we set $weight\ decay = 1e-5$, and we set it to 0 for the information extraction task. For information extraction, $batch\ size = 4$ due to memory limit and we use all data in one iteration for adequate training samples in each epoch. The performance are reported on 20,000 random test samples for pre-training task and 700 given test data (200 in test set of TestA, 500 in test set of TestB) for information extraction task.

4.3 Experimental Results

we adopt tree edit distance (TED) based accuracy [5,17,18] for information extraction task.

In terms of evaluation metrics, we adopt Acc (Accuracy) for information extraction task at the request of the organizer, it is calculated as, $(TP+TN)/(P+N)$, where TP(TN) stands for the number of positive(negative) samples predicted to be right, and P(N) denotes the number of total positive(negative) samples. There are also some works adopting tree edit distance (TED) based accuracy [5,17,18] for information extraction task. The evaluation metric for pseudo-OCR pre-training task is ANLS (Average Normalized Levenshtein Similarity) which is an edit-distance based metric.

Overall, we fine-tune the whole model on VD and the training task is pseudo-OCR. After fine-tuning the model for the information extraction task, the model participates in the IEMPD task evaluation of CHIP 2022.

The result of pseudo-OCR task test is shown in Tabel 3. Since the pre-training task is relatively simple, there is no special data processing, we directly feed the image into the model, and calculate the cross-entropy loss between the output text of the model and the label text. After training, we use ANLS to evaluate the reading ability of the model. From the reading failure cases, we can find that the model's reading failure is mainly due to the difficulty in distinguishing Chinese and other language punctuation marks and other contents.

Table 3. Average Normalized Levenshtein Similarity (ANLS) scores on VD. We set the time cost of Donut as the standard 100%.

Model	ANLS	Time
Donut [7] (Before fine-tuning)	73.7	100%
Donut (fine-tuned)	97.8	100%
Ours (384*384 input)	**98.3**	13.0%
Ours (224*224 input)	96.2	**10.9%**

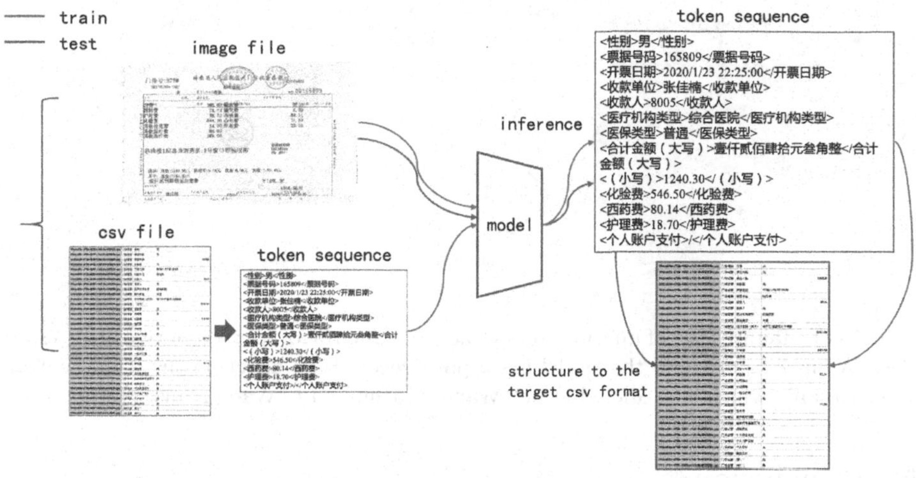

Fig. 4. The data pipline.

For the IEMPD task evaluation of CHIP 2022, the result is shown in Tabel 4. Note that there is not any data augmentation used in this task. There is also not any data pre-processing or post-processing. However, it is highly possible to achieve better results with appropriate augmentation, training hyperparameters, and other tricks. Due to the generality of the scheme, it can be fine-tuned by adding other open source Chinese document images. We choose not to do these due to time constraints, which indirectly shows that our scheme has a very high upper bound and is very scalable. The data pipline is shown in Fig. 4.

Table 4. Accuracy (Acc) scores on IEMPD task in CHIP 2022.

Model	Acc (test set of TestA) %	Acc (test set of TestB) %
Donut [7]	54.1	50.7
Ours	**59.0**	**62.0**

For this result, we believe that the end-to-end models can hardly perform well directly. We think that adding sophisticated pre-processing and post-processing can significantly improve the results, but we don't do that. The model itself of course has its own problems. Through the observation of the validation set, we think that the most important error is caused by the low accuracy of the model in recognizing Chinese characters. We have almost no time to combine the results of the two tasks. In Fig. 5, the model mistakenly recognizes the character. Such cases still abound. The main reason for this phenomenon is that the open source model in [7] is mainly trained in English, Korean and other foreign languages, and Chinese is less. In finetune, the data size is also small, and many Chinese characters may not appear in the training set. Due to the generality of the scheme, it can be fine-tuned by adding other open source Chinese document images.

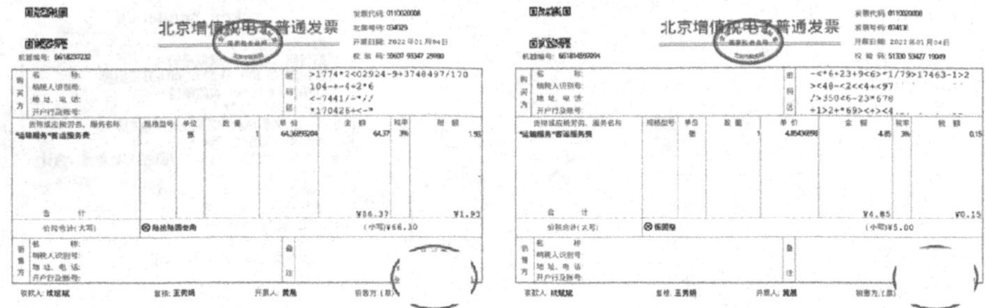

Fig. 5. The failure case of information extraction. The review person of two invoices are both Wang Xiujuan, and the model has a poor recognition effect on the Chinese character "Juan", which is predicted to be "Wang Xiushu" and "Wang Xiuru" respectively.

5 Conclusion

The method proposed in this paper implements visual parsing from document images in an end-to-end manner, which is a multi-modal scheme. Actually, we are not the first to do this, but previous fine-tuning work is hard to make multilingual models perform well in specific language scenarios such as Chinese, and the inference time of the model is too long, making it difficult to use in industry.

By fine-tuning the model on the original pre-training task, we allow the model to fully learn Chinese character features on VD while effectively retaining the gains from the initial large-scale multilingual pre-training. To speed up inference, we reduced the input size of the model but found that it did not perform as well, which we believe is due to the fact that the model was given large images and optical characters in the original pre-training task. Large image input in pre-training limits the model to handle small images int the downstream tasks. We use the small image input in the fine-tuning of the pseudo-OCR task, and the experiment shows that the model is competent for the visual parsing of small document images. Finally, in the evaluation TestB, the acc score of our model is 0.6202 in the IEMPD task in CHIP 2022, ranking second in open source code.

Acknowledgements. This work was supported by the Infinity Security, Hangzhou, China.

References

1. Baek, J., et al.: What is wrong with scene text recognition model comparisons? dataset and model analysis. In: Proceedings of the IEEE/CVF International Conference on Computer Vision, pp. 4715–4723 (2019)
2. Baek, Y., Lee, B., Han, D., Yun, S., Lee, H.: Character region awareness for text detection. In: Proceedings of the IEEE/CVF Conference on Computer Vision and Pattern Recognition, pp. 9365–9374 (2019)

3. Hong, T., Kim, D., Ji, M., Hwang, W., Nam, D., Park, S.: Bros: a pre-trained language model focusing on text and layout for better key information extraction from documents. In: Proceedings of the AAAI Conference on Artificial Intelligence, vol. 36, pp. 10767–10775 (2022)
4. Hwang, W., et al.: Post-ocr parsing: building simple and robust parser via bio tagging. In: Workshop on Document Intelligence at NeurIPS 2019 (2019)
5. Hwang, W., Lee, H., Yim, J., Kim, G., Seo, M.: Cost-effective end-to-end information extraction for semi-structured document images. arXiv preprint arXiv:2104.08041 (2021)
6. Hwang, W., Yim, J., Park, S., Yang, S., Seo, M.: Spatial dependency parsing for semi-structured document information extraction. arXiv preprint arXiv:2005.00642 (2020)
7. Kim, G., et al.: Ocr-free document understanding transformer. In: Avidan, S., Brostow, G., Cissé, M., Farinella, G.M., Hassner, T. (eds.) Computer Vision - ECCV 2022, ECCV 2022. LNCS, vol. 13688, pp. 498–517. Springer, Cham (2022). https://doi.org/10.1007/978-3-031-19815-1_29
8. Lewis, M., et al.: Bart: denoising sequence-to-sequence pre-training for natural language generation, translation, and comprehension. arXiv preprint arXiv:1910.13461 (2019)
9. Li, J., Xu, Y., Lv, T., Cui, L., Zhang, C., Wei, F.: Dit: self-supervised pre-training for document image transformer. arXiv preprint arXiv:2203.02378 (2022)
10. Liu, Chang, Z., et al.: Information extraction of medical materials: an overview of the track of medical materials medocr. In: Health Information Processing (2022)
11. Liu, Chang, Z., et al.: Medocr: the dataset for extraction of optical character recognition elements for medical materials. J. Med. Inf. **43**(12), 4 (2022)
12. Liu, Z., et al.: Swin transformer: Hierarchical vision transformer using shifted windows. In: Proceedings of the IEEE/CVF International Conference on Computer Vision, pp. 10012–10022 (2021)
13. Majumder, B.P., Potti, N., Tata, S., Wendt, J.B., Zhao, Q., Najork, M.: Representation learning for information extraction from form-like documents. In: Proceedings of the 58th Annual Meeting of the Association for Computational Linguistics, pp. 6495–6504 (2020)
14. Xu, Y., et al.: Layoutlmv2: multi-modal pre-training for visually-rich document understanding. arXiv preprint arXiv:2012.14740 (2020)
15. Xu, Y., Li, M., Cui, L., Huang, S., Wei, F., Zhou, M.: Layoutlm: pre-training of text and layout for document image understanding. In: Proceedings of the 26th ACM SIGKDD International Conference on Knowledge Discovery & Data Mining, pp. 1192–1200 (2020)
16. Yim, M., Kim, Y., Cho, H.-C., Park, S.: SynthTIGER: synthetic text image GEneratoR towards better text recognition models. In: Lladós, J., Lopresti, D., Uchida, S. (eds.) ICDAR 2021. LNCS, vol. 12824, pp. 109–124. Springer, Cham (2021). https://doi.org/10.1007/978-3-030-86337-1_8
17. Zhang, K., Shasha, D.: Simple fast algorithms for the editing distance between trees and related problems. SIAM J. Comput. **18**(6), 1245–1262 (1989)
18. Zhong, X., ShafieiBavani, E., Jimeno Yepes, A.: Image-based table recognition: data, model, and evaluation. In: Vedaldi, A., Bischof, H., Brox, T., Frahm, J.-M. (eds.) ECCV 2020. LNCS, vol. 12366, pp. 564–580. Springer, Cham (2020). https://doi.org/10.1007/978-3-030-58589-1_34
19. Zong, L.L., et al.: Overview of technology evaluation dataset for medical multimodal information extraction. J. Med. Inf. **43**(12), 6 (2022)

Improving Medical OCR Information Extraction with Integrated Bert and LayoutXLM Models

Lianchi Zheng[1,2], Xiaoming Liu[1,2,3](✉), Zhihui Sun[1,3], and Yuxiang He[1,3]

[1] Zhongyuan University of Technology, Zhengzhou 450007, China
ming616@zut.edu.cn

[2] Henan Key Laboratory on Public Opinion Intelligent Analysis, Zhengzhou 450007, China

[3] Zhengzhou Key Laboratory of Text Processing and Image Understanding, Zhengzhou 450007, China

Abstract. Currently, medical records in most hospitals are paper-based and rely on manual input, but with the advancements in OCR and NLP technologies, it is now possible to convert such records into electronic and structured formats. In this paper, we explore the CHIP2022 evaluation task 4 and compare the performance of two pre-training models: Bert without additional coordinate information and LayoutXLM with additional coordinate information. We apply a selection and regularization process to refine the results and evaluate our framework's accuracy through a list in Ali Cloud Tianchi. Our results demonstrate that our framework achieved good performance.

Keywords: Bert · LayoutXLM · Regularization

1 Introduction

As the COVID-19 outbreak continues worldwide, hospitals are facing increasing medical pressure. Among the challenges that hospitals face daily, dealing with numerous types of medical invoices not only creates complexity but also adds pressure to hospital staff. In everyday life, individuals encounter invoices regularly, and hospitals issue a considerable number of invoices in the course of their operations. Tedious invoice management processes and tremendous manual labor [1] costs have become major concerns. Moreover, the vast majority of medical invoices used in hospitals is paper-based, which is prone to damage and leads to data and economic losses. With artificial intelligence advancing at an unprecedented pace, an increasing number of invoice recognition systems based on deep learning technology, such as Baidu's OCR identification system and Tencent's OCR identification system, are emerging in the market. This paper aims to digitize medical invoices and use OCR technology to extract invoice information accurately and efficiently. Such innovation can reduce invoice processing time, save labor costs in parallel, increase the accuracy of information records, and enable unified management in medication and other aspects, overhauling medical staff's responsibility, and preventing

B. Tang et al. (Eds.): CHIP 2022, CCIS 1773, pp. 164–173, 2023.
https://doi.org/10.1007/978-981-99-4826-0_16

the occurrence of non-standard medical advice. Ultimately, it protects patients' rights and interests, avoids disputes and accidents, and safeguards the interests of medical staff [2].

Existing frameworks for automated critical field extraction tasks can be expensive and prone to errors, particularly when extracting data from medical and invoice forms following OCR recognition. Medical invoices comprise structured data or information fields such as vendor name, vendor address, invoice date, invoice number, invoice total, Goods and Services Tax (GST) number, and list of items. Developing an automated key field extraction framework that can extract this relevant data can significantly raise an organization's productivity by minimizing error-prone and manual work [3].

The MedOCR task in CHIP2022 presents complex scenarios, such as outpatient and inpatient invoices, which feature numerous extracted content, irregular layout formats, and low image quality. As a result, they are prone to text recognition errors. Additionally, labeling OCR data is also challenging. To address these difficulties, we propose a two-stage approach. Firstly, we use an advanced OCR model to extract the picture's text and then perform text sequence annotation as the later named entity recognition's annotation data to extract information. We also correct some text errors based on the label's text. Finally, we use the Bert [4] model for named entity recognition to obtain the desired information. Additionally, we directly select the advanced LayoutXML [5] multimodal model that includes coordinate information for direct end-to-end recognition. Ultimately, we combine the two recognition results to obtain the final recognition results effectively. To validate our model's effectiveness, we participated in Alibaba Cloud Tianchi and achieved an accuracy rate for each item, as shown in Table 1.

2 Related Work

Deep learning has achieved great success in text detection and recognition for the OCR domain. However, extracting key information from documents is a more critical task, and there are currently three types of existing models: raster-based, graph-based, and end-to-end.

- **Raster-based.** Raster-based methods convert images into a raster representation vector based on image pixels, which is then inputted into deep learning networks to learn and extract key information. However, the relationship between the texts in the document is not only affected by the text sequence but also by the layout distribution of each text. To address this issue, Katti et al. proposed the Chargrid method [6], which maps document images into a character-level 2D grid representation. One-hot encoding is adopted for each character grid, and the vector representation is used as input for Chargrid-Net. The method uses an encoder-decoder CNN network structure for text box detection and semantic segmentation of key information. Similarly, Zhao et al. developed the CUTIE method [7] to address the inability of NLP technology alone to process layout information among various texts in a document. CUTIE maps the document image to a raster vector representation that retains the spatial position relation of each text and uses two types of CNN models to extract key information.

- **Graph-based.** The graph structure-based method regards the document picture as a graph structure composed of text slices, and uses a neural network model to learn the relationship between text slices to extract the key information content of the document. Liu, Xiaojing, et al. [8] pointed out that the traditional NER method BiLSTM-CRF could not make use of the layout information between text slices in document images. This paper proposes to use a graph convolutional neural network to learn the semantic information and layout information of text slices, and construct a fully connected graph structure by treating text slices as points and inter-text relations as edges. The graph vector representation of each text slice is learned by using the graph convolutional neural network, which is then spliced with the Word2Vec vector of each text token in the text slice and input into the BiLSTM-CRF network for key information extraction of documents and images. The entire model is optimized by text slice classification task and IOB sequence classification task.

  Xu, Yiheng, et al. [9] pointed out that pre-training models have achieved great success in the field of NLP but lacked the utilization of layout and layout information, making them unsuited for the task of extracting key information from documents and images. Therefore, the LayoutLM model was proposed, which uses BERT (a powerful pre-training model in the NLP field) as the backbone network. To make use of the layout and layout information, a 2D position vector representation is introduced, obtaining vectors of the two-point annotations of each text slice (horizontal and vertical coordinates in the upper-left corner and the lower-right corner) through index tables in the horizontal and vertical directions, respectively. Optionally, visual vector representations of slices can be added to provide more information. Since BERT can fundamentally be viewed as a fully connected graph network, we also classify LayoutLM as a graph structure-based technique.

  Later, LayoutLm-like pre-training models such as Lambert [10] appeared, which obtained SOTA structure on key information extraction tasks of documents and images, proving the powerful ability of deep learning models based on large corpora and large models.
- **End-to-end.** End-to-end refers to the direct extraction of the key information content of a document from the original input image. Guo, He et al. [11] highlighted that information extraction technologies based on detection and recognition processes may be affected by slight positional offsets. To overcome these problems, the EATEN method was proposed, which directly extracts the key information content of the document from its original input image. Zhang, Peng et al. [12] noted that existing key information extraction methods rely on multiple independent tasks, such as text detection, text recognition, and information extraction, which are not supervised and learned from each other. As a solution, the authors proposed an end-to-end network model called TRIE that simultaneously learns from the aforementioned three tasks.

Based on the existing work, this paper utilizes the LayoutXLM model with multi-modal task combination and directly applies the Bert model for named entity recognition. By comparing and exploring the combined results, it aims to achieve an improved outcome.

3 Proposed Framework

The framework proposed in this study is based on the BERT model, which employs a mask language model (MLM) and a layoutXML model to implement BioNER tasks. By integrating the two frameworks, we aim to improve the accuracy of recognition, particularly for inputs with poor eigenvalues, and to obtain more reasonable and accurate recognition results after matching. It is worth noting that we did not introduce additional annotated data in this mission prediction; instead, we directly obtained results from NER annotations.

3.1 Main Model

The BERT model is a highly potent yet simple concept model, constructed by stacking the simplest Transformer structures to form the core architecture of the model as depicted in Fig. 1. During pre-training, it is necessary to employ the Masked Language Model (MLM) because under standard conditions, the model can only be trained from either left-to-right or right-to-left directions. The MLM technology is introduced to predict target words in complex sentences. To address the limitation of the model, some tokens are replaced with a random percentage of [mask], which is then predicted. To mitigate any adverse effects of [mask], the following operation is performed during pre-processing:

1. It has an 80% probability of being replaced with a normal [mask], for example: My heart is broken—— > My heart is [mask].
2. It has a 10% chance of being replaced with a random word, for example: My heart is broken—— > My heart is lonely.
3. There is a 10% chance that the original word will remain the same, for example: My heart is broken—— > My heart is broken. We also add task-specific class tokens ([CLS]) to the input of the BERT model.

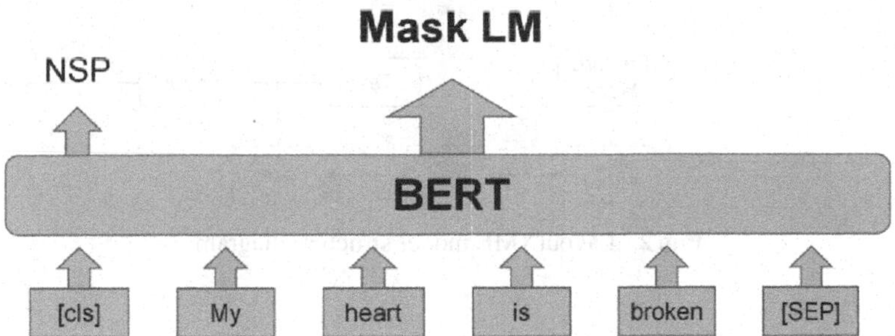

Fig. 1. Main structure of BERT model

The LayoutXLM model is designed with a multimodal transformer architecture, similar to the LayoutLMv2 [13] framework. The model accepts information from three different modes, including text, layout and image, which are coded as the text embedding layer, layout embedding layer and visual embedding layer respectively. After text and image embeds are concatenated, layout embeds are added to give model input. We use this model to realize the recognition of medical forms, and for key value extraction, one of the most critical tasks in form understanding, similar to FUNSD, this task is defined as two sub-tasks, namely semantic entity recognition and relationship extraction, task description. We're using semantic entity recognition.The core framework of the model in Fig. 2.

In the Semantic Entity Recognition (SER) subtask, the descriptive methods are as follows:

Given A rich text document A, get the token sequence t = {t_0, t_1..., t_n}, where each token can be expressed as t_i = (w, (x_0, y_0, x_1, y_1)), w is the token text, and (x_0, y_0, x_1, y_1) is the spatial coordinate position of the text in the document. Define the class of all semantic entities as C = {c_0, c_1,... c_m}. The semantic entity recognition task requires the model tag to extract all defined semantic entities and classify them into correct categories, that is, to find the function Fser:(A, C) - >, where E is the semantic entity set predicted by the model:

$$\varepsilon = \left\{\left(\left\{t_0^0, \cdots, t_0^{n0}\right\}, c_0\right), \cdots, \left(\left\{t_k^0, \cdots, t_k^{nk}\right\}, c_k\right)\right\}$$

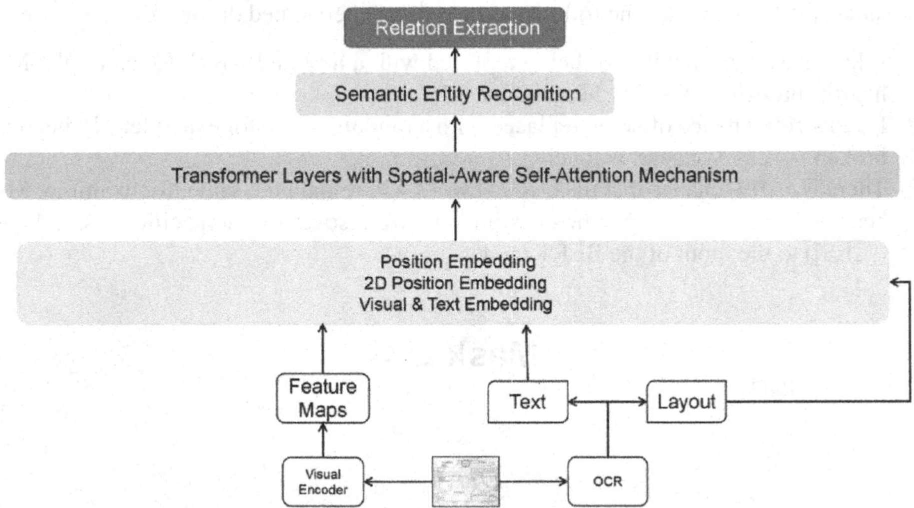

Fig. 2. LayoutXML model structure diagram

4 Experiment

4.1 Datasets

The experiment was conducted using the OCR identification of electronic medical paper documents (ePaper) task dataset of the CHIP2022 Evaluation Task 4 medical invoice. The dataset employed in this study encompasses 1000 samples for recognition training.

This dataset comprises 200 discharge summary invoices, 200 medicines invoices, 200 outpatient invoices, and 400 hospitalization invoices, all of which are real-world images, together with labeled results. The identification evaluation comprises two distinct lists – TestA and TestB. TestA lists 200 real-world images with corresponding marked results for identification assessment. TestB, on the other hand, lists 500 real-world images with matching marked results. It is worth noting that each class has different tags that need to be extracted.

To transform the given data into trainable structural data, we annotated the dataset while exploring the similarity threshold of tag and text matching. Subsequently, we performed experiments individually using the Bert and LayoutXLM models. Finally, we combined the results of both models to evaluate the overall model performance.

4.2 Image OCR Recognition and Error Correction

In this study, we employed PaddleOCR [14] to recognize each image. The recognition result comprised sentence-based text content together with their corresponding coordinate information. We then corrected any identification errors using single word similarity in order to avoid the labeling effect being impacted by excessive identification errors. We found the corresponding relationship between each label and the sentence in each photo. Taking the length of the label as the window and a step size of one for matching, we computed the average value as the similarity between the contents of the window and the label. We subsequently set a threshold for similarity at 0.66. Any similarity scores exceeding this value were considered as errors. In such cases, the contents of the window were changed to match the label values.

4.3 Data Labeling

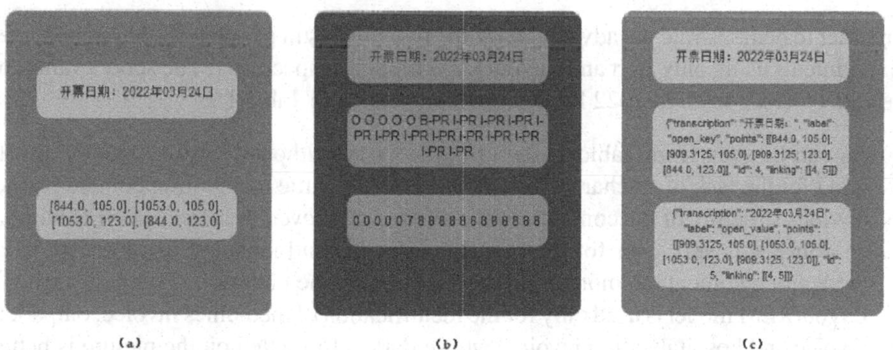

Fig. 3. (a)Sample one of the original data. (b)Sample of BERT's NER annotation. (c)Sample annotation of SER for LayoutXLM.

– Bert uses named entity recognition (NER) to identify the key information, so it needs to use BIO annotation. The code is used for annotation. The original data is shown in Fig. 3(a), and the annotated data is shown in Fig. 3(b). Specific implementation of BIO annotation:

1. Read the annotations given in the dataset.
2. Read the recognition result of each image and divide it into single words.
3. Match each sample word and get the result.
4. Structured storage.

- Since the LayoutXLM training data is in the unit of sentences, the identified results are divided into sentences and then compared with the sentence label sentence by sentence. Sometimes coordinates need to be merged and split. The marked data is shown in Fig. 3(c). It's a label for each entity but it's actually still a BIO tag on the inside but it's just a different representation on the outside. Specific implementation of annotation:

   1. Read the text and coordinates after image recognition.
   2. Error correction of identification results.
   3. Compare according to the labels to obtain the labels of each coordinate frame.
   4. Structured storage.

4.4 Setting

- Bert adopts AdamW as the optimizer, lr is 2e-5, linear attenuation of learning rate is adopted, and the maximum number of training rounds is 96. Use transformers 4.7.0 and Pytorch 1.10.1 to structure the training model and push it to the huggingface community [15] for invocation.
- LayoutXLM employs AdamW as an optimizer, lr 2e-5, linear attenuation of learning rate, maximum number of training rounds of 200, and training with paddle 2.3.2.

4.5 Experimental Results

In order to demonstrate the advantages of the two models in parallel, we have conducted experiments using only Bert and LayoutXLM models respectively. The score evaluation results of TestB in CHIP2022 Evaluation 4 are shown in Table 1.

- As can be seen from Table 1, the effect of NER without coordinates is relatively good for the task of discharge summary, which has little recognition content but not obvious structure of the contents on the picture. However, the effect of NER without coordinates is very poor for the outpatient invoice and inpatient invoice with more recognition content but more structured content on the picture.
- LayoutXLM model is used only for the identification of medicines invoice, outpatient invoice and hospitalization invoice, whose data is formatted on the picture is better, but for the categories of discharge summary invoice with lower structured data but less identification content, the effect will be worse.
- Based on the above comparison, we combine the results of the two models through regularization query, and it can be concluded that each index of the two models has improved, which is 22.19% higher than that of Bert and 2.7% higher than that of LayoutXLM. Therefore, this method is effective.

Table 1. The score evaluation results of TestB in CHIP2022 Evaluation 4

Model	Evaluation Metrics	Score
Bert	CYXJ-Acc	0.8094
	GYFP-Acc	0.5705
	MZFP-Acc	0.1276
	ZYFP-Acc	0.1433
	Acc	0.2486
LayoutXLM	CYXJ-Acc	0.5162
	GYFP-Acc	0.6378
	MZFP-Acc	0.3437
	ZYFP-Acc	0.4337
	Acc	0.4435
Bert + LayoutXLM	CYXJ-Acc	0.8094
	GYFP-Acc	0.7384
	MZFP-Acc	0.3495
	ZYFP-Acc	0.4237
	Acc	0.4705

5 Conclusion

This paper explores the relationship between Bert and LayoutXLM for OCR information extraction tasks based on the CHIP2022 evaluation task 4. The results are refined through regularization and splicing to obtain better results. To label data in BIO format, we extrapolated word-to-word similarity to sentence-to-sentence similarity. Our findings indicate that Bert achieves higher accuracy in extracting information from discharge summary invoice, presumably because there are fewer entities to be identified, whereas LayoutXLM accuracy decreases due to coordinate information errors. For the other three types, the accuracy is higher in LayoutXLM since their coordinate information is relatively regular in the picture. Lastly, we regularized the integrated results and modified them to make them more reasonable. In the evaluation TestB, CYXJ-Acc, GYFP-Acc, MZFP-Acc, ZYFP-Acc, and Acc were 0.8094, 0.7384, 0.3495, 0.4237, and 0.4705, respectively, ranking our paper third in open source code.

Acknowledgment. We gratefully thank the anonymous reviewers for their helpful comments and suggestions. This study was supported partly by the National Natural Science Foundation of China (NSFC No.62076167), Ministry of Education industry-school cooperative education project (Grant No. 201902298016), and Key Research Project of Henan Higher Education Institutions (Granted No. 23A520022).

References

1. Shi, S., Cui, C., Xiao, Y.: An invoice recognition system using deep learning. In: 2020 International Conference on Intelligent Computing, Automation and Systems (ICICAS). pp. 416–423. IEEE (2020)
2. Yao, X., Sun, H., Li, S., Lu, W.: Invoice detection and recognition system based on deep learning. Secur. Commun. Netw. **2022**, 1–10 (2022)
3. Baviskar, D., Ahirrao, S., Kotecha, K.: Multi-layout unstructured invoice documents dataset: a dataset for template-free invoice processing and its evaluation using AI approaches. IEEE Access **9**, 101494–101512 (2021)
4. Devlin, J., Chang, M.-W., Lee, K., Toutanova, K.: Bert: Pre-training of deep bidirectional transformers for language understanding. arXiv preprint arXiv:1810.04805 (2018)
5. Xu, Y., et al.: Layoutxlm: multimodal pre-training for multilingual visually-rich document understanding. arXiv preprint arXiv:2104.08836 (2021)
6. Katti, A.R., et al.: Chargrid: towards understanding 2d documents. arXiv preprint arXiv:1809.08799 (2018)
7. Zhao, X., Niu, E., Wu, Z., Wang, X.: Cutie: learning to understand documents with convolutional universal text information extractor. arXiv preprint arXiv:1903.12363 (2019)
8. Liu, X., Gao, F., Zhang, Q., Zhao, H.: Graph convolution for multimodal information extraction from visually rich documents. arXiv preprint arXiv:1903.11279 (2019)
9. Xu, Y., Li, M., Cui, L., Huang, S., Wei, F., Zhou, M.: Layoutlm: Pre-training of text and layout for document image understanding. In: Proceedings of the 26th ACM SIGKDD International Conference on Knowledge Discovery & Data Mining, pp. 1192–1200 (2020)
10. Garncarek, R., et al.: Lambert: Layout-aware language modeling for information extraction. In: Document Analysis and Recognition–ICDAR 2021: 16th International Conference, Lausanne, Switzerland, 5–10 September 2021, Proceedings, Part I. Springer, Cham, pp. 532–547 (2021)
11. Guo, H., Qin, X., Liu, J., Han, J., Liu, J., Ding, E.: Eaten: entity-aware attention for single shot visual text extraction. In: 2019 International Conference on Document Analysis and Recognition (ICDAR), pp. 254–259. IEEE, (2019)
12. Zhang, P., et al.: Trie: end-to-end text reading and information extraction for document understanding. In: Proceedings of the 28th ACM International Conference on Multimedia, pp. 1413–1422 (2020)
13. Xu, Y., et al.: Layoutlmv2: multi-modal pre-training for visually-rich document understanding. arXiv preprint arXiv:2012.14740 (2020)
14. Li, C., et al.: Pp-ocrv3: More attempts for the improvement of ultra lightweight ocr system. arXiv preprint arXiv:2206.03001 (2022)
15. Wolf, T., et al.: Transformers: state-of-the-art natural language processing. In: Proceedings of the 2020 Conference on Empirical Methods in Natural Language Processing: System Demonstrations, pp. 38–45 (2020)
16. Chen, Y.-C., et al.: UNITER: Universal image-text representation learning. In: Vedaldi, A., Bischof, H., Brox, T., Frahm, J.-M. (eds.) ECCV 2020. LNCS, vol. 12375, pp. 104–120. Springer, Cham (2020). https://doi.org/10.1007/978-3-030-58577-8_7
17. Shi, B., Bai, X., Yao, C.: An end-to-end trainable neural network for image-based sequence recognition and its application to scene text recognition. In: Arxiv (2015)
18. Mori, S., Suen, C., Yamamoto, K.: Historical review of OCR research and development. Proc. IEEE **80**(7), 1029–1058 (1992)
19. Ming, D., Liu, J., Tian, J.: Research on Chinese financial invoice recognition technology. Arxiv Pattern Recogn. Lett. **24**(1), 489–497 (2003)

20. Zong, H., Lei, J., Li, Z., et al.: Overview of technology evaluation dataset for medical multimodal information extraction. J. Med. Inf. **43**(12), 2–5+22 (2022)
21. Liu, L., Chang, D., Zhao, X., et al.: MedOCR: the dataset for extraction of optical character recognition elements for medical materials. J. Med. Inf. **43**(12), 28–31 (2022)
22. Liu, L., Chang, D., Zhao, X., et al.: Information extraction of medical materials: an overview of the track of medical materials MedOCR. In: Health Information Processing: 8th China Conference, CHIP 2022, Hangzhou, China, 21–23 October 2022, Revised Selected Papers. Springer, Singapore (2022)

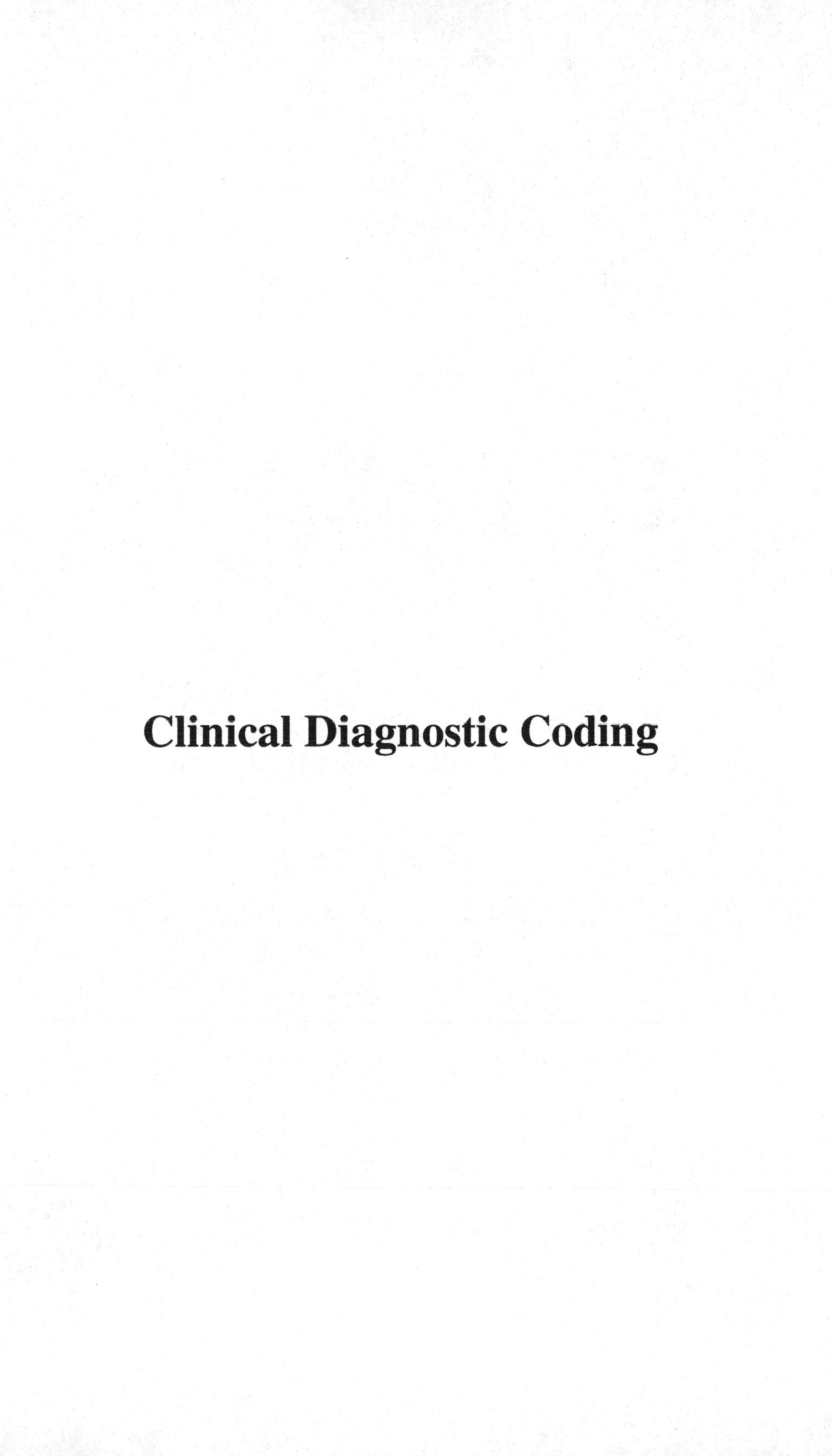

Clinical Diagnostic Coding

Overview of CHIP 2022 Shared Task 5: Clinical Diagnostic Coding

Gengxin Luo[1], Bo Kang[2], Hao Peng[1], Ying Xiong[1], Zhenli Lin[3], and Buzhou Tang[1,4](✉)

[1] Harbin Institute of Technology (Shenzhen), Shenzhen, China
luo_hai@foxmail.com, 903871772@qq.com, xiongying@hit.stu.edu.cn
[2] Yidu Cloud (Beijing) Technology Co. Ltd., Beijing, China
bo.kang@yiducloud.cn
[3] Department of Ophthalmology, Shenzhen University General Hospital, Shenzhen, China
13728901687@163.com
[4] Pengcheng Laboratory, Shenzhen, China
tangbuzhou@gmail.com

Abstract. The 8th China conference on Health Information Processing (CHIP2022) released 5 shared tasks related to Chinese medical information processing. Among them, the fifth task is about clinical diagnosis coding, which demands assigning the standard medical diagnostic words to the possible medical concepts in the visiting information. A total of 10 teams participated in the task and finally submitted 19 sets of results. This task takes the average F1 score as the final evaluation index, and the highest F1 score among all submission reaches 0.6908.

Keywords: Clinical Diagnosis Encoding · Natural Language Processing · Pre-trained Language Model

1 Introduction

In the field of healthcare, a large amount of medical text data is stored in the form of electronic medical records (EMR). EMRs including various medical information of patients contain important statistical value. However, EMRs are often recorded by medical workers during disease diagnosis. Due to the differences in the information systems of hospitals and the individual habits of recorders, this leads to different expressions and quality of the same disease in different EMRs, which brings difficulties to the follow-up processing work [1].

The clinical diagnosis coding technology can automatically assign one or more standard medical diagnostic words according to the medical-related concepts hidden in the medical record samples. The generation of these standard diagnostic words will effectively improve the processing efficiency of the subsequent statistical or other tasks on EMRs. With the development of natural language processing technology, more and more text processing tasks have been effectively solved, including the processing of

B. Tang et al. (Eds.): CHIP 2022, CCIS 1773, pp. 177–184, 2023.
https://doi.org/10.1007/978-981-99-4826-0_17

medical texts. In this context, how to effectively implement clinical diagnostic coding technology with the help of natural language processing technology becomes a hot topic in recent related research.

The 8th China conference on Health Information Processing (CHIP2022) released five shared tasks related to Chinese medical and health information processing [2], of which the fifth task is about clinical diagnosis coding. This task requires participants to code the Chinese EMRs, that is, given a series of patient information, they are required to give the standard diagnostic words corresponding to this medical record. Among them, the standard diagnostic words are based on the vocabulary of "National Clinical Version 2.0 of Classification and Codes of Diseases" as a standard. The data set used in this task is provided by Yidu Cloud (Beijing) Technology Co., Ltd. Each training sample contains various medical information of the patient and the corresponding standard diagnostic words. The sample data is shown in Table 1.

Table 1. An example of data sample.

Visiting information (or standard diagnostic words)	Content
Discharge diagnosis	Left kidney tumor, Hypertension
Surgery name	Transabdominal partial left nephrectomy + use of artificial intelligence assisted therapy plus charges
Preoperative diagnosis	Renal tumor of both kidney
Postoperative diagnosis	-
Admission diagnosis	Left kidney tumor, Hypertension
Drug name	Alanyl glutamine, Lactulose, Celecoxib, Budesonide, Palonosetron, Flurbiprofen, Chymotrypsin glucose (19%)
Medical advice	Disposable oxygen inhalation tube type ot-mi-100, Disposable sterile syringe with needle 1ml (kdl/control), Routine urinalysis (urinalysis + urine sediment) (instrumental method), Oxygen nebulizer inhalation, Urological care routine, Biochemical routine (emergency) (electrolytes + liver and kidney function + blood glucose + cardiac + crp) tests
Standard diagnostic words	Renal neoplasms; primary hypertension

2 Related Work

Clinical diagnosis coding is to process disease diagnosis and treatment information of patients. And it is an important part of medical record information management. Today, clinical diagnosis coding has become one of the most important basic for scientific and informational management of hospitals. It has been increasingly used in evaluating medical quality and efficiency, designing clinical pathway plans, hospital evaluation, disease diagnosis grading, rational drug use monitoring, etc.

Currently, the International Classification of Diseases (ICD), an internationally unified disease classification method developed by WHO, is the most influential and popular among various classification schemes [3]. Larkey and Croft used three classifiers in machine learning to automatically code the discharge summary of inpatients, and they assigned a unique ICD code to each sample [4]. Kavuluru et al. proposed a multi-label classification method based on electronic health records (EHR) [5]. Early machine learning methods ignored the context dependence of text, and these methods are not effective enough for today's complex and highly redundant clinical diagnostic information. With the rapid development of deep learning technology, deep neural network has gradually been applied in the field of medical information processing. Huang et al. used RNN and CNN for ICD automatic coding [6]. They also found that on clinical diagnostic coding tasks, methods based on deep learning generally outperformed those based on machine learning. Xie et al. proposed a LSTM network based on a tree-sequence structure and transformed the automatic encoding problem into a semantic matching problem [7]. Compared with traditional machine learning methods, deep learning technology can better utilize the semantic information contained in texts.

Since 2018, the China conference on Health Information Processing (CHIP) has released several tasks related to medical and health information processing [8, 9], which has promoted the development of related research in the interdisciplinary fields of medical information and artificial intelligence. In CHIP2019, the clinical terminology standardization task was released, which requires the standardization of the original surgical words given in the Chinese electronic medical records and mapping to the corresponding standard surgical words in the standard vocabulary [10]. The clinical diagnosis coding task proposed in this paper is a further extension of the clinical terminology standardization task. The difference between the two tasks is that the clinical diagnosis coding task does not mark the medical terms that need to be standardized in the data set, but only provides various medical information in the medical record samples and demands directly generating relevant standard medical diagnostic words, which brings challenges to this task.

3 Assessment Data

The CHIP2022 shared task 5 data set was compiled and marked by a professional medical team based on professional experience, and was provided by Yidu Cloud (Beijing) Technology Co., Ltd. The training set contains 2,700 samples, of which each sample contains medical information and its corresponding one or more standard diagnostic words based on the vocabulary of "National Clinical Edition 2.0 of the Classification and Code of Diseases". The medical information includes discharge diagnosis, surgery name, preoperative diagnosis, postoperative diagnosis, admission diagnosis, drug name and medical advice. The test set contains 337 medical information samples, and the contestants are required to give their corresponding standard diagnostic words according to the given medical information. In addition, there are 278 different standard diagnostic words in the training set, and each of the standard diagnostic words in the test set have appeared among these 278 words [11]. Table 2 shows the statistical results of each medical information and diagnostic standard words in the data set.

Table 2. Statistical information of dataset.

Statistical objects	Training set	Test set
Average length of discharge diagnosis	24.84	25.19
Average length of surgery name	11.61	12.15
Average length of preoperative diagnosis	4.49	4.48
Average length of postoperative diagnosis	3.76	4.00
Average length of admission diagnosis	21.62	21.67
Average length of drug name	89.69	91.06
Average length of medical advice	917.21	934.70
Average length of standard diagnostic word	18.33	18.43
Average number of standard diagnostic word	3.1	2.8

4 Assessment Results

4.1 Evaluation Index

The evaluation index used in clinical diagnostic coding task include precision rate (P), recall rate (R) and F1 score. The F1 score is used as the ranking index. The calculation methods of related index are as follows:

$$P = \frac{\textit{The number of true predicted standard words}}{\textit{The number of predicted standard words}}$$

$$R = \frac{\textit{The number of true predicted standard words}}{\textit{The number of true standard words}}$$

$$F1 = \frac{2 \times P \times R}{P + R}$$

4.2 Analysis of Methods

The dominant approaches in this task are introducing pre-trained language models and improving the models based on them, pre-processing the data based on prior knowledge, and post-processing the output standard diagnostic words. The participants used a variety of pre-trained language models, including BERT [12], a standard model for bidirectional encoding of transformers, Chinese RoBERTa for Chinese texts [13], and long text pre-trained language models such as Longformer [14] and BigBird [15]. In addition, some teams also adopted other ideas, such as rule matching based on feature words.

The 1st ranked team first combined medical knowledge and human experience to pre-process the data based on knowledge graphs for term normalization, filtering, and labeling. Then they used the pre-trained model BERT and made improvements to it by adding a Value-Pooling structure [16], which was added to output a matrix instead of a vector and could be better suited for the task of outputting multiple variable number of categories. Meanwhile, they used Focal Loss and preprocessed labels directly related to the target to enhance the loss weights of their corresponding labels to optimize the loss.

The 2nd ranked team analyzed various types of consultation information, performed feature selection, and then formed a set of text pairs with all features and each standard diagnostic word. Then they performed binary classification on each pair by a pre-trained model to determine whether the standard diagnostic word in the text pair matched the medical information text. Moreover, they divided the original dataset into five folds for cross-validation.

The 3rd ranked team constructed a special drug dictionary with a total of 4 feature drug dictionaries, including chemotherapy drugs, targeted drugs, endocrine drugs, and immune drugs. And, they established corresponding diagnostic rules based on medical feature words, groups and combinations, and then matched diagnostic criteria words by the established rules.

4.3 Analysis of Results

The results submitted by the 10 participating teams are analyzed and the mean F1 score is 0.5186, the maximum 0.6908 and the median 0.5730. Table 3 presents information on the best results submitted by each of the top three teams, including the method description and F1 score.

In this shared task, most of the teams used pre-trained language models, and the basic idea of these methods is to match text pairs with the form <clinical diagnosis information, standard diagnostic words> through the pre-trained model. The top one team analyzed the characteristics of this task and concluded that the general approach based on pre-trained models using the vector corresponding to the [CLS] labels directly as output is more suitable for multi-category tasks where each sample belongs to only one category. Whereas, in clinical diagnostic coding task each sample corresponds to multiple non-exclusive and variable number of categories. Therefore, they proposed a Value-Pooling structure so that the model directly outputs a matrix where each vector in the matrix corresponds to a criterion word in the diagnostic criteria word list, thus achieving better results. Alternatively, some teams have used methods other than language models, such as rule-based matching models, which have also achieved good results.

Table 3. The assessment results of the top three teams

Rank	Competition participants	Method description	F1 score
1	Alibaba Cloud	pre-trained language model BERT, Value-Pooling structure, loss optimization	0.6908
2	Beijing Academy of Artificial Intelligence	pre-trained language model Chinese RoBERTa, feature filtering, cross validation	0.6609
3	National University of Defense Technology	feature dictionaries on drug, rule matching based on feature words	0.6581

The test set used in this task contains 337 samples and 178 different standard diagnostic words. Figure 1 counts the number of selected standard diagnostic words in the test set and the number of correct predictions for them by different teams. As it can be seen from the figure, the distribution of diagnostic criteria words is not uniform.

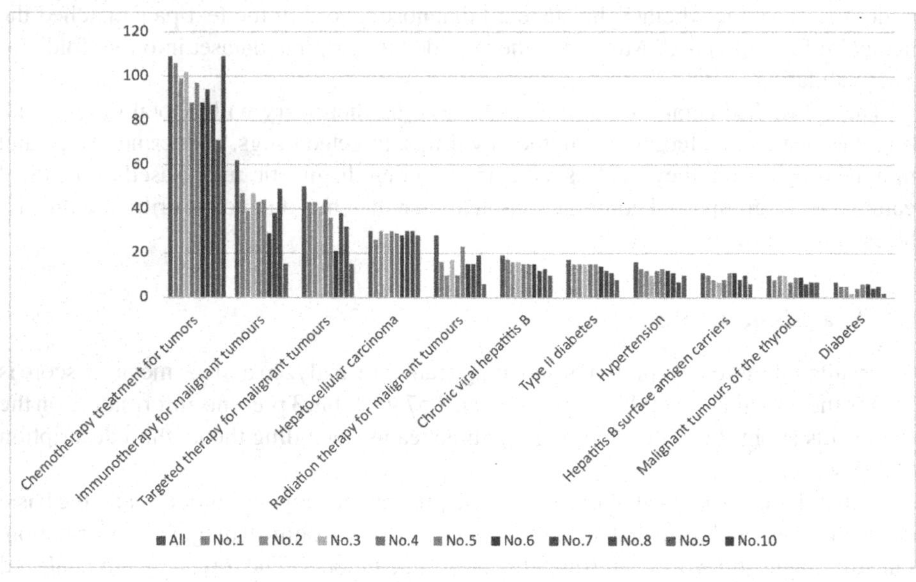

Fig. 1. Correctly predicted sample number of each team for some labels.

As for error analysis, we choose different combinations of teams and integrate their models. And the integrated model reaches the best performance when choosing the top five teams and setting the voting threshold as 2, which means when there are two or more models output a standard diagnostic word x on the same sample then we consider the integrated model output this standard word x. The highest F1 score the integrated model can reach is 0.7231, about 3% points higher than the top one model.

In addition, some standard diagnostic words in the test set are never output by any team's model. Those words are shown in Table 4. A potential reason is the frequency of their appearance in the test set is very low.

Table 4. The standard diagnostic words not output by any participant's model

The words not output by any model		
Palliative chemotherapy	Carcinoma in situ of the colon	Compound cancer
Post-operative endocrine therapy for tumors	Personal history of malignant tumors of the breast	Operation not performed for other reasons
Anemia	Personal history of malignancy	Symptomatic treatment
Malignant tumor of the upper lobe of the lung	Non-toxic mononodular goiter	Malignant tumor of the lower outer quadrant of the breast
Malignant tumor of the breast, lower	Malignant tumors of the upper and lower lobes of the lung	Hypertensive disease grade 2 (high risk)
Multiple malignant tumors of the thyroid gland	Malignant tumor of the posterior bladder wall	Post-operative incision infection
Malignant tumor of the lower inner quadrant of the breast	Endocervical malignancy	Malignant tumor of the breast, lateral
Autologous peripheral blood stem cell mobilization	Lymphocytic thyroiditis	Malignant tumor of the upper inner quadrant of the breast

5 Conclusion

With the informatization process of hospital management, classification and normalization of diseases and surgery becomes an import sessions of medical record management. Due to the rapid development of natural language processing technology, different methods were proposed to realize clinical diagnostic coding.

This paper gives an overview of CHIP2022 shared task: clinical diagnostic coding. In total, 3037 Chinese medical information samples are released for this task, including 278 different standard diagnostic words. A total of 10 teams submitted the results. The top one model was structurally improved based on a pre-trained language model, and its F1 score reached 0.6908. Most of the other participating teams also introduced pre-trained language models, and these methods generally achieved better results than methods that did not introduce pre-trained models.

The CHIP2022 shared task 5 provides a reliable data set and experimental results for the clinical diagnosis coding task. The analysis results show that the prediction effect of most of the team's model teams is relatively poor for diagnostic standard words that contain semantic information and have containment and similarity relations. In future research work, how to better distinguish such fine-grained diagnostic coding is the key to further improving the performance of clinical diagnostic coding models.

Acknowledgements. This study is partially supported by National Key R&D Program of China (2021ZD0113402), National Natural Science Foundations of China (62276082), Major Key Project of PCL (PCL2021A06), Pilot Project in 5G + Health Application of Ministry of Industry and Information Technology & National Health Commission (5G + Luohu Hospital Group: an Attempt to New Health Management Styles of Residents).

References

1. Sun, W., Cai, Z., Li, Y., et al.: Data processing and text mining technologies on electronic medical records: a review. J. Healthc. Eng. (2018)
2. Zong, H., Lei, J., Li, Z., et al.: Overview of technology evaluation dataset for medical multimodal information extraction. J. Med. Indform. **43**(12), 2–5+22 (2022)
3. World Health Organization. The ICD-10 classification of mental and behavioural disorders: clinical descriptions and diagnostic guidelines. World Health Organization (1992)
4. Larkey, L.S., Croft, W.B.: Combining classifiers in text categorization. In: Proceedings of the 19th Annual International ACM SIGIR Conference on Research and Development in Information Retrieval, pp. 289–297 (1996)
5. Kavuluru, R., Rios, A., Lu, Y.: An empirical evaluation of supervised learning approaches in assigning diagnosis codes to electronic medical records. Artif. Intell. Med. **65**(2), 155–166 (2015)
6. Xie, P., Xing, E.: A neural architecture for automated ICD coding. In: Proceedings of the 56th Annual Meeting of the Association for Computational Linguistics (Volume 1: Long Papers), pp. 1066–1076 (2018)
7. Huang, J., Osorio, C., Sy, L.W.: An empirical evaluation of deep learning for ICD-9 code assignment using MIMIC-III clinical notes. Comput. Methods Programs Biomed. **177**, 141–153 (2019)
8. Medical Health and Bioinformation Processing Committee of Chinese Information Society of China. In: The 6th China conference on Health Information Processing (CHIP2020) (2022). http://www.cips-chip.org.cn/2020/eval1
9. Medical Health and Bioinformation Processing Committee of Chinese Information Society of China. In: The 7th China conference on Health Information Processing (CHIP2021) (2022). http://www.cips-chip.org.cn/2021/eval1
10. Huang, Y., Jiao, X., Tang, B., et al.: Overview of CHIP 2019 shared task: clinical terminology standardization. Chin. J. Inform. **35**(3), 94–99 (2021)
11. Luo, G., Kang, B., Peng, H., et al.: Overview of the clinical diagnostic coding technology assessment dataset and baseline model. J. Med. Inform. **43**(12), 10–15 (2022)
12. Devlin, J., Chang, M.W., Lee, K., et al.: Bert: pre-training of deep bidirectional transformers for language understanding. arXiv preprint arXiv:1810.04805 (2018)
13. Liu, Y., Ott, M., Goyal, N., et al.: Roberta: a robustly optimized bert pretraining approach. arXiv preprint arXiv:1907.11692 (2019)
14. Beltagy, I., Peters, M.E., Cohan, A.: Longformer: the long-document transformer. arXiv preprint arXiv:2004.05150 (2020)
15. Zaheer, M., Guruganesh, G., Dubey, K.A., et al.: Big bird: transformers for longer sequences. Adv. Neural. Inf. Process. Syst. **33**, 17283–17297 (2020)
16. He, Y., Wang, C., Zhang, S., et al.: KG-MTT-BERT: Knowledge Graph Enhanced BERT for Multi-Type Medical Text Classification. arXiv preprint arXiv:2210.03970 (2022)

Clinical Coding Based on Knowledge Enhanced Language Model and Attention Pooling

Yong He(✉), Weiqing Li, Shun Zhang, Zhaorong Li, Zixiao Ding, and Zhenyu Zeng

Alibaba Group, Hangzhou, China
{sanyuan.hy,liweiqing.lwq,changchuan.zs, zhaorong.lzr,dingzixiao.dzx,zhenyu.zzy}@alibaba-inc.com

Abstract. Clinical coding is obtaining a standard ICD code based on the patient's electronic medical record (EMR) information, including diagnosis, procedure, drug list, order, etc. It is essential in the medical record information management of the hospital. However, the medical record data have problems such as low quality, insufficient data, full of non-standardized jargon, irrelevant order information, and unbalanced data distribution, which result in poor performance of clinical coding. This task is a multi-label classification problem. Based on the medical pre-trained language model and our medical knowledge engineering (MetaMed KE), we proposed a Value-Level Attention Pooling (VLAP) to build a clinical diagnostic coding framework for Chinese electronic medical records. The framework includes three components: preprocessing module, the model, and the postprocessing module. Compared to existing algorithms, our framework dramatically improves the generalization ability and accuracy in the case of insufficient data and class unbalance. Thus, our method provides a reliable automatic solution for clinical coding in hospital medical record information management.

Keywords: Clinical Coding · Electronic Medical Record · Text Classification · Pre-trained Language Model · Knowledge Enhanced

1 Background

1.1 Clinical Coding

Clinical coding has become one of the crucial bases for the scientific and informational management of hospitals. It is vital in evaluating medical quality and efficiency, designing clinical pathway plans, disciplines ranking, hospital evaluation, diagnosis and grading, infectious disease reporting, DRGs payment, rational drug use, etc. Clinical diagnostic coding, a subtask of clinical coding, is based on the relevant information in electronic medical records to give an ICD code and name in the standard diagnostic catalog, such as "Classification and Code of Diseases National Clinical V2.0".

Y. He and W. Li—Equal Contribution.

B. Tang et al. (Eds.): CHIP 2022, CCIS 1773, pp. 185–205, 2023.
https://doi.org/10.1007/978-981-99-4826-0_18

Currently, clinical diagnosis coding for Chinese electronic medical records in hospitals still relies on manual coding, which has problems of insufficient low accuracy, low efficiency, high cost, and inconsistent criteria. With the rapid development of artificial intelligence, technologies for clinical diagnostic coding using machine learning and deep learning emerge in an endless stream. However, most of the existing work based on short medical texts is difficult to process the redundant information in Chinese electronic medical records, which have low-quality, full of non-standardized terms, and irrelevant order information. In addition, there are some troubles of insufficient information. For example, the data richness in a hospital is inadequate. A patient may have multiple diagnoses. The completeness of the diagnosis information in the electronic medical record is insufficient. Therefore, it needs to be inferred by combining the doctor's order information, medicine list, and medical knowledge.

We built an automated clinical diagnosis coding framework for Chinese electronic medical records to solve the above problem. First, this framework uses the normalization algorithm to process the non-standard input terms, short medical text preprocessing for low-quality data, medical order classification and labeling, etc. [19] Then, it applies MetaMed KE to obtain the medical knowledge behind the input terms and integrate them into the input. Secondly, we propose the Value-Level Attention Pooling (VLAP) method based on the pre-trained medical language model. Next, the model is trained under the guidance of target-related knowledge. Finally, a post-processing module is designed to ensure the reliability of model prediction results. In short, we provide a practical framework for clinical diagnosis coding, which provides a reliable automatic solution for hospital information management.

1.2 ICD-10

The International Classification of Diseases (ICD) [2] is an internationally unified disease classification method formulated by the World Health Organization (WHO). Diseases are classified, making them an ordered group and represented by a coded system. Currently, the most widely used in the world, including China, is the 10th version, called ICD-10. The diagnosis names in the original ICD-10 are in English. The National Health Commision and the National Healthcare Security Administration have translated, optimized, expanded, etc., on this basis to form the Chinese version of ICD-10 [3], including more than 40,000 Article diagnosis, ICD10 national clinical version, and ICD10 national medical insurance version. Over time, version upgrades will also be carried out, such as "Disease Diagnosis Code ICD-10 National Clinical Version 1.1", "Disease Diagnosis Code ICD-10 National Clinical Version 2.0", "Disease Diagnosis Code ICD-10 National Medical Insurance Version 1.0", "Disease Diagnosis Code ICD-10 National Medical Insurance Version 2.0", and so on. Some diseases have regional characteristics. For example, there are differences in the incidence, number of patients, and distribution of the same diagnosis between China's eastern and western regions. At the same time, the development trend and process of certain diseases in different areas are inconsistent, such as developed regions having advantages in technology, capital, talent, and the number of patients. As a result, certain diseases in developed areas develop more refinedly. Therefore, different regions will also expand and optimize the basic national version.

1.3 Difference Between What Doctors Write and Standard Coding

In clinical diagnosis coding, the information includes the diagnosis name written by the doctor, so why not directly use the diagnosis name recorded by the doctor as the standard diagnosis code? There are the following reasons:

1) There are non-standard terms for the diagnosis written by doctors. For example, "Autoimmune Disease (Hepatitis)" needs to be mapped to the ICD-10 code "K75.400" and the name "Autoimmune Hepatitis".
2) In some cases, the doctor uses the name of the procedure performed this time as a diagnosis because many patients are admitted to the hospital only for a specific surgical procedure, or this surgical procedure is the primary resource consumption for this admission, such as "Percutaneous Nephrolithotomy".
3) There may be omissions, mistakes, overwriting, or missed diagnosis codes, etc. Some patients suffer from multiple diseases in a single admission and need to be treated across various departments. The doctor who writes the diagnosis may only be in the department of the primary diagnosis, so the diagnosis of other departments may be missed. For example, the diseases treated by the patient include "Hypertension" and "Benign Prostatic Hyperplasia" in hospital admission, but there may be only "Prostatic Hyperplasia".
4) It may need to be processed with other information, such as the procedure and medication. If a doctor writes "Mucosa-Associated Lymphoid Tissue Extranodal Marginal Zone Lymphoma (Malt Lymphoma)" and targeted therapies are given, then the standard diagnostic name is "Malignant Tumor Targeted Therapy".
5) The diagnosis may change as the patient stays in the hospital. If the admission diagnosis is "Left Breast Mass, Palpable at 9 o'clock", the standard diagnosis is "Mammary Tumor, Inner Side".
6) There are complications in the diagnosis, such as "Type 2 Diabetes with Multiple Complications" and "Type 1 Diabetes with Coma". Some diagnoses need to be refined, such as "Type 1 Diabetes" and "Type 2 Diabetes", "Hypertension Grade 1", "Hypertension Grade 2", and "Hypertension Grade 3".
7) The doctor's writing and medical record coding guidelines are inconsistent. Doctors predispose the patient's disease, while the standard diagnosis code tends to the classification system of diagnosis, which includes not only the disease but also treated information, such as complications, procedure, treatment process, etc.

The rest of the paper is organized as follows. Section 2 is a review of related works and techniques. Section 3 describes the task and challenges. Section 4 is the introduction of our framework in detail. Section 5 reports the performances of our model in the dataset and investigates hyperparameter effects and multiple ablation studies to further the understanding of the model. Section 6 is the conclusion and future directions.

2 Related Works

Clinical Coding is a very general and basic medical text-mining task, and many studies have been in this area. He et al. [4] built a model called KG-MTT-BERT, which applied knowledge graphs to enhance the pre-trained model for the multi-type medical text classification problem. This paper [5] introduces the use of different machine learning and deep learning techniques in solving this problem and evaluates and compares the performance and effect of these techniques in different environments. Song et al. [6] proposed a latent feature generation framework to improve the prediction performance of rare diagnostic codes without compromising the performance of common codes, exploiting the hierarchy of ICD codes and using a novel recurrent structure reconstructs encoding-related keywords to generate semantically meaningful features for zero-shot diagnostic encoding. This work [7] built a machine learning model BERT-XML for large-scale automatic ICD encoding based on the recently popular unsupervised pre-training language model BERT. Li et al. [8] proposed a multi-filter residual convolutional neural network (MultiResCNN) for ICD coding. This paper [9] provided a new label attention for ICD auto-encoding, which can not only deal with different lengths of text fragments related to ICD encoding but also with the interdependence of these text fragments. At the same time, a hierarchical federated learning mechanism is also proposed, which extends the label attention model to exploit the hierarchical relationship between diagnostic codes to optimize the scheme. This research [10] proposed a hyperbolic and co-occurrence graph representation method (HyperCore) to solve the ICD-10 automatic coding problem using the code hierarchy and co-occurrence. This paper [11] proposes a hierarchical deep learning model with an attention mechanism to assign ICD diagnosis codes given a written diagnosis automatically. Authors of this paper [12] proposed a BERT-based clinical terminology standardization method. This method uses the Jaccard similarity algorithm to select candidate words from the standard term set. Then it matches the original and candidate words based on the BERT model to obtain standardized results.

This task belongs to natural language processing (NLP), and the most commonly used is the pre-trained language model. There are three common modes. The first is a bidirectional language model represented by BERT [13] for natural language understanding (NLU). The second is GPT3 [14] for natural language generation (NLG) is the unidirectional language model. The third type is the mixed language model for unified text-to-text-format represented by T5 [15].

Medical care is a knowledge-intensive industry emphasizing authority, rigor, accuracy, and explainability, so medical knowledge is a critical input source. DKPLM [16] and KG-MTT-BERT [4] applied knowledge to enhance the pre-trained language model. This paper also uses DKPLM as part of our model.

3 Problem Description

3.1 Task Information

Clinical diagnostic coding integrates, summarizes, and processes various information in electronic medical records written by doctors to form one or more standard diagnostic codes and corresponding diagnostic names. The medical record information based on it includes basic patient information, admission records, surgical procedure, discharge records, and various diagnosis names written by doctors (such as admission diagnosis, preoperative diagnosis, postoperative diagnosis, and discharge diagnosis). The standard diagnostic codes and names come from the existing diagnostic code catalogs. The general diagnosis of Western medicine is based on ICD-10, such as "Disease Diagnosis Code ICD-10 National Clinical Edition 2.0", "Disease Diagnosis Code ICD-10 National Medical Insurance Edition 2.0", "Disease Diagnosis Code ICD-10 National Medical Insurance Version 1.0", etc. There are many versions of standard diagnostic codes in China, and different provinces and cities will expand on the basic ICD-10 version issued by the country. Because many diseases are regional, different places and medical institutions may use different standard versions. For example, The ICD-10 used by a hospital in Hangzhou differs from that used in Guangzhou.

3.2 Data Description

1) Data Details. Medical care is an industry with a very high data density. From the patient's admission to the discharge to medical insurance payment, medical research, etc., in this series of medical activities, data will be generated around the patient, as shown in Fig. 1.

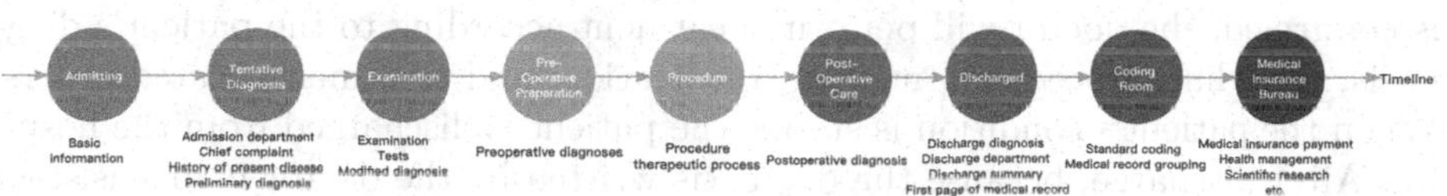

Fig. 1. Medical Data Generation Timeline

Diagnosis: From the perspective of medical knowledge, medical care is a knowledge-intensive industry emphasizing authority, rigor, accuracy, and interpretability. Diagnosis is the most critical information in medical knowledge, and much medical knowledge revolves around disease or diagnosis, which is the heart of the medical knowledge graph. Although the word-formation of the diagnosis is brief, there are many types and amounts of knowledge behind it. As shown in Fig. 2.

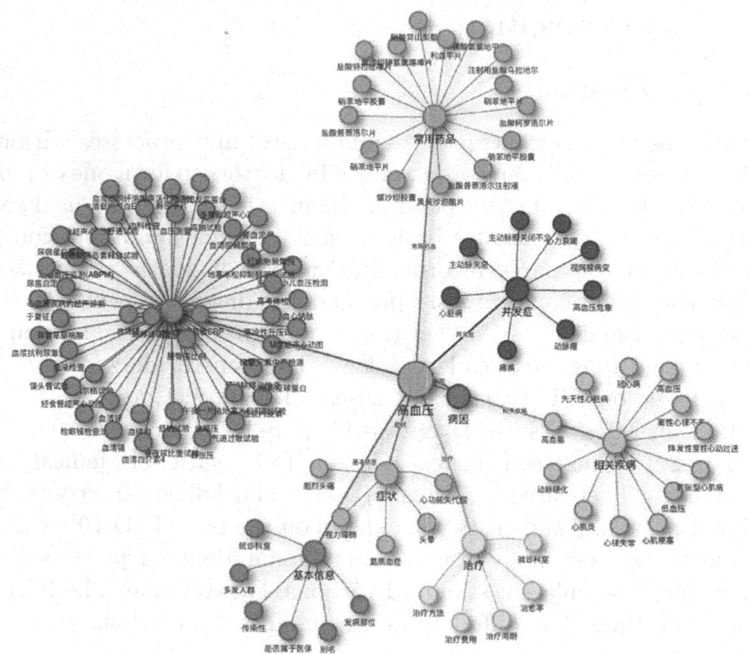

Fig. 2. Diagnosis-Centric Medical Knowledge Graph

From the perspective of medical activities, diagnosis is the carrying point and the most critical information in a series of medical activities centered around patients. When the patient is admitted to the hospital, the doctor will diagnose based on the inspection information and laboratory tests. Once the diagnosis is confirmed, the doctor will perform treatment according to the patient's diagnosis, including procedures, nursing, medication, and treatment-related orders. When the patient's condition is stable, the patient is discharged from the hospital. After discharge, because the diagnosis written by the doctor is inconsistent with the definitive diagnosis, the hospital's coders will carry out a standard diagnosis code for this admission. The information relied on in the standardization process includes lots of information generated by patients during the admission process, especially the diagnosis written by doctors, procedures, doctor's orders, medicines, etc. Subsequent medical activities are carried out around standard diagnostic codes, such as medical insurance payment, medical research, and health management. The details are shown in Fig. 3.

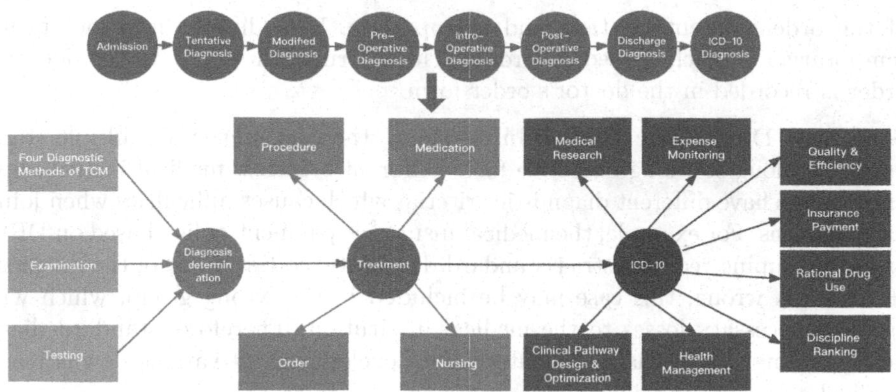

Fig. 3. Diagnosis-Centric Medical Activities

During the patient's admission, the diagnoses involved in the medical records include admission diagnosis, preoperative diagnosis, postoperative diagnosis, and discharge diagnosis. There may be one or more of each diagnosis. As the patient stays in the hospital, some changes will occur in the diagnosis, such as revision, addition, merger, etc. The diagnostic standards generally use ICD-10 as the standard version, and different regions expand and optimize it, so there are subtle differences, such as Beijing, Guangdong, Zhejiang, and so on. Although there is a standard diagnostic version, doctors may have their writing habits when recording, or the EMR system of the hospital uses its diagnosis catalog, or doctors cannot find corresponding code in the standard diagnostic catalog, resulting in a large number of non-standardized names for the diagnoses written by doctors.

Procedure: When doctors treat a patient, they impose specific procedures for treatment. A therapeutic procedure involves accessing the body's interior by making an incision on the surface of the patient's body. When doctors perform a procedure on a patient, they keep detailed records, including the specific procedure name, the detailed process, and the patient's condition. There are also standardized catalogs for procedures, such as ICD-9-CM-3, which will be expanded in different regions, resulting in subtle differences. Although there is a standard catalog of procedures, there are the same problems as when recording diagnoses.

Medication: During treatment, the doctor will choose the corresponding medication according to the diagnosis and condition, including therapeutic, surgical, nursing, and auxiliary drugs. The drug information consists of the name, dosage, and specification, which are recorded in the patient medication record.

Order: During the patient's stay in the hospital, the doctor will give the patient instructions on diet, medication, examination, laboratory tests, consumables, etc., according to the condition and treatment. An order is a medical instruction issued by a doctor in treatment. The information of the doctor's order consists of the order content, a start, and a stop time. It is divided into long-term, temporary, and backup medical orders. The information related to the doctor's order is recorded in the doctor's order form.

Standard Diagnostic Codes: In medicine, the coexistence of multiple standards is a long-standing objective fact. Different systems, medical institutions, and regions have different diagnostic criteria, which causes difficulties when joint data analysis. For example, the medical insurance payment policy based on DRG or DIP grouping requires strict standard diagnostic codes. If one of the diagnostic codes is wrong, this case may be included in the wrong group, which will cause unnecessary losses to the medical institution. Therefore, standard diagnostic coding is essential to facilitate the development of various downstream medical activities in medical care.

2) Dataset Description. In the dataset of CHIP2022, the sources include admission diagnosis, preoperative diagnosis, procedure, postoperative diagnosis, discharge diagnosis, drug name list, and doctor's order, and the target is the standard diagnosis, using "Category of Diseases and Codes National Clinical Edition 2.0" as the standard diagnostic catalog. The set of dataset targets is a subset of the standard catalog. Some examples are shown in Fig. 4.

We conduct a brief analysis of the dataset. The training set includes 2700 samples, a total of 278 labels. The test set has a total of 337 samples without labels. The training set has a class imbalance problem. For example, the label with the largest number of samples is "For Tumor Chemistry Treatment Course", with 912 samples. The second number label is "Malignant Tumor Immunotherapy", which is halved to 440. The label with the fewest samples only has four samples, involving 159 labels with four samples. The statistics show in Fig. 5(a). The size of the label set of each sample is 1 6, the size is unfixed, and its distribution is shown in Fig. 5(b). There are 2700 samples with procedures and 1534 samples without procedures. Most samples are related to tumors and cancers, so the dataset focuses on tumors and is subdivided. The solution needs to be granular to deal with insufficient data.

<table>
<tr><th>出院诊断</th><th>手术名称</th><th>术前诊断</th><th>术后诊断</th><th>入院诊断</th><th>药品名称</th><th>医嘱</th><th>target</th></tr>
<tr><td>右肾癌 pt2an0m0 高血压</td><td>经腹右肾部分切除术+使用人工智能辅助治疗加收（si)</td><td>左 右 双肾 肾肿瘤</td><td></td><td>右肾癌 高甘油三酯血症 高尿酸血症 高血压</td><td>ω-3鱼油脂肪乳 丙氨酰谷氨酰胺 乳果糖 地西泮 塞来昔布。. .</td><td>"3m透气型透明敷料(固定导管)9546hp.10*11.5cm. x线计算机体层(ct)扫描加收(使用螺旋扫描) 一次性使用吸氧管ot-mi-100型.小号.(零感) . . .</td><td>肾恶性肿瘤;原发性高血压</td></tr>
<tr><td>食管胃结合部癌 pt4an3bm1 iv期</td><td>腹腔镜辅助贲门癌根治术（贲门癌切除+d2淋巴结切除+食管空肠r-y吻合）+肝脏结节切除术</td><td>食管胃结合部肿物伴消化道出血</td><td>食管胃结合部肿物伴消化道出血</td><td>重度贫血 食管胃结合部癌 ct3n2m0</td><td>ω-3鱼油脂肪乳 丙氨酰谷氨酰胺 中/长链脂肪乳(c8-24) 呋塞米 地西泮 . . .</td><td>"(可来福)输液接头||01c-c3300(可来福)：100个/盒 3m透明敷料(固定导管)(明尼苏达)||1679.10*11.5cm 3m透气型透明敷料(固定导管)9546hp.10*11.5cm. cvc护理 一体式吸氧管(舒氧宝)ty-xyg-22(宁波天益) . . .</td><td>食管胃连接处恶性肿瘤;胃淋巴结继发恶性肿瘤</td></tr>
</table>

Fig. 4. Examples of the Dataset

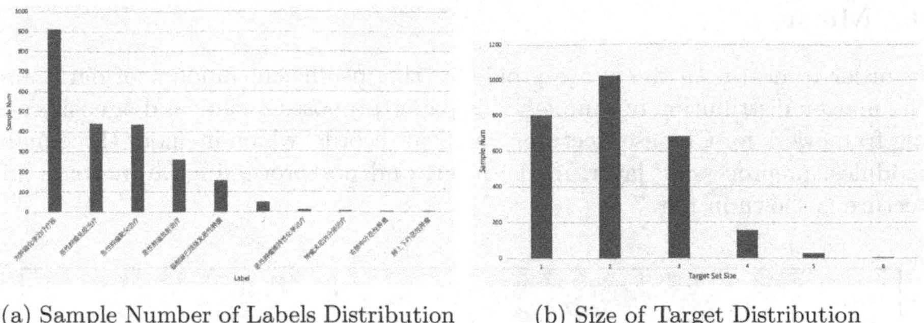

(a) Sample Number of Labels Distribution (b) Size of Target Distribution

Fig. 5. Distribution

3.3 Task

We extract this task into a computable problem and obtain one or more definitive diagnoses for this admission based on various medical record information of a patient to form a set of definitive diagnoses, which is a typical multi-label text classification problem. Its input consists of various medical clinical text information, and its target is an ICD-10 diagnosis set.

According to the above dataset description, admission diagnosis, preoperative diagnosis, procedure, postoperative diagnosis, discharge diagnosis, drug name list, and doctor's order are input fields, and the target is an ICD-10 code. Each field is a set of terms (input terms are not standardized, and output terms are standard diagnostic names). The problem is: input multiple types of sets, each set element is a term, and output a set that belongs to a multi-label classification problem based on multiple types of short text terms. This process is highly specialized but very suitable for abstraction as a modeling problem. Its inputs and outputs are shown in Fig. 6.

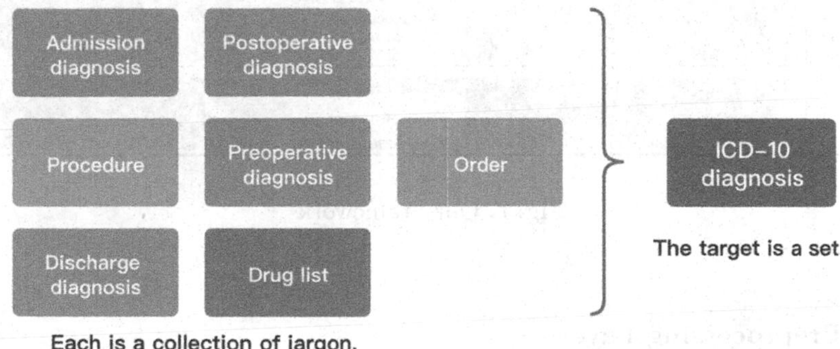

Fig. 6. Problem

4 Method

In order to deal with the above problems, the insufficient amount of data, and the uneven distribution of samples, this paper proposes a clinical diagnosis coding framework for Chinese electronic medical records, which includes three main modules: preprocessing layer, model layer, and postprocessing layer. Its architecture is shown in Fig. 7.

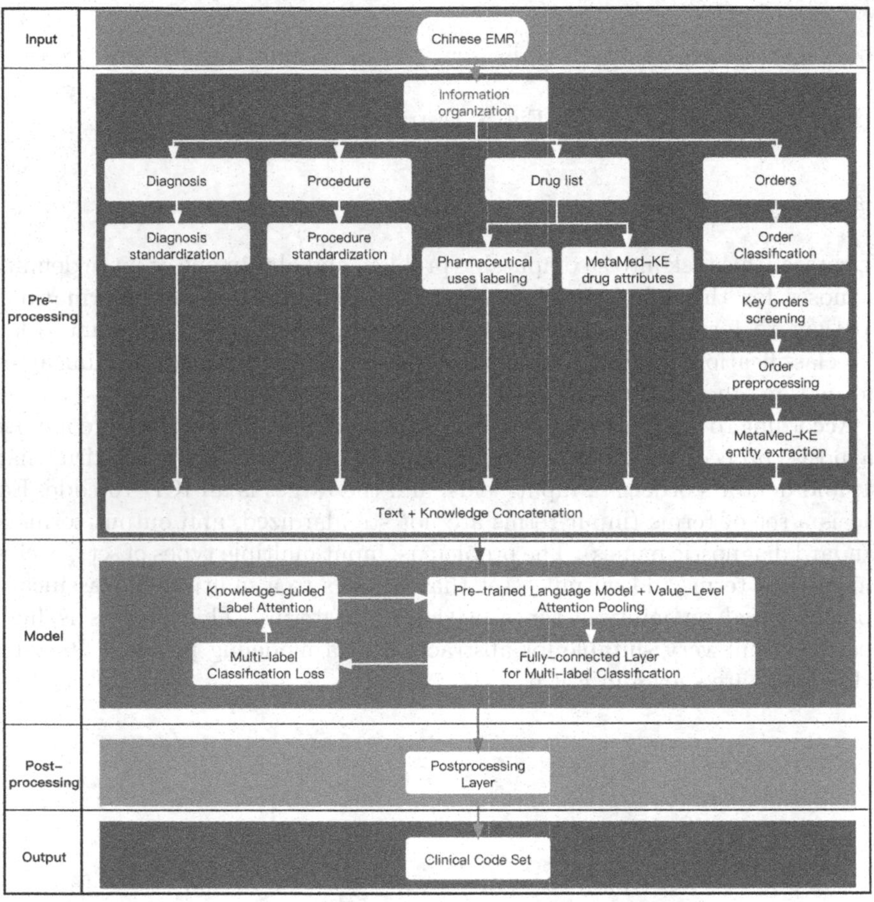

Fig. 7. Our Framework

4.1 Preprocessing Layer

According to Chinese electronic medical records, the information is organized into several fields, including diagnosis, procedure, drug list, and doctor's orders. The original data is processed through the following data preprocessing and enhancement to mine the medical knowledge behind the data.

1) Diagnosis and Procedure Name. The input diagnoses and procedures contain many unstandardized terms, such as "Hypertension Grade 1" and "Hypertension Grade I". These terms with the same meaning are normalized to the same name.

Terminology Standardization: Non-standardized diagnostic and procedural terms were mapped to the "Classification and Codes of Diseases National Clinical Version 2.0" and the "Classification of Procedures National Clinical Version 2.0" by our term normalization algorithm, such as "Invasive Carcinoma of the Left Breast" standardized to "Malignant Tumor of the Breast", "Carcinoma of the Left Ureter" standardized to "Malignant Tumor of the Ureter", and "Hysteroscopic Myomectomy" standardized as "Myomectomy". Then, concatenate the normalized term string with the unnormalized term string as the output string of this step.

2) Drug Name. Drug information is very useful for the diagnostic labels, especially key drugs related to diagnosis.

Pharmaceutical Uses Labeling: Use our drug use knowledge base to mark each drug and select the critical use drugs related to the target, mainly including "chemotherapy", "targeted therapy", "immunotherapy", "endocrine therapy", "diabetes drug", "hypertension drugs", etc. We are connecting important label names to drug names to enhance the algorithm for identifying different types of malignant tumors and other vital diseases, such as "Cisplatin" for chemotherapy, "Nimotuzumab" for targeted therapy, "Goserelin" for endocrine therapy, "Camrelizumab" for immunotherapy, "Metformin" for "type 2 diabetes", "Captopril" for a high blood pressure, etc.

Drug Superordinate Attributes: It is difficult for the diagnostic coding model to learn valuable coding knowledge from fewer data for other medicines with names but no attributes and uses. Therefore, we applied MetaMed KE to extract the superordinate attributes for non-anticancer drugs, including the ingredients, uses, and other attributes. After that, some attributes are filtered by constructing an attribute set of target-related to prevent noise. Afterward, for each sample, TF-IDF is used to mine the expressions of all MetaMed KE superordinate concept terms that frequently appear in the sample and finally splice it with the drug name as the output string of the sample in this step. For example, the superordinate concept terms of "Aspirin" are "Salicylic Acid and ts Derivatives", "Analgesics", "Nervous System Drugs", and "Chemicals". After filtering through the target-related attribute set, "Analgesic Drug" and "Nervous System Drug" are reserved.

3) Order. The doctor's order contains a lot of information, and some of the information plays a crucial role in the diagnosis coding. Screening the target-related information from the doctor's order is the guarantee of the algorithm result.

Order Classification: First, utilize our medical item classification model to automatically classify the doctor's order text sentences, including "examination", "inspection", "drugs", "nursing", "consumables", "surgery", "chemotherapy", "targeted therapy", "endocrine therapy", "immunotherapy", "radiation therapy", and "none".

Key Orders: We screen for some important order categories, including "examinations", "tests", "drugs", "surgery", "chemotherapy", "targeted therapy", "endocrine therapy", "immunotherapy", "radiation treatment" and annotate these filtered orders. For example, "Checkout and discharge today" is classified as "none", it will be filtered and not used. "Chemotherapy Care [Order]" is a key order because of containing "chemotherapy treatment". "Xeloda is 50 tablets in total, 2 mornings and 3 nights, and d1 night -d11 early [order]" is also a critical order because of containing "chemotherapy drugs".

Order Preprocessing: For the key doctor's orders after the screening, preprocessing is required. Use our order preprocessing model to filter out useless characters in the order text. For example, "Xeloda is 50 tablets in total, 2 mornings and 3 evenings, d1 night-d11 early [order]" is processed to "Xeloda"; "Simple mastectomy under general anesthesia tomorrow, sentinel lymph node biopsy [order]" is processed to "Simple Mastectomy" and "Sentinel Lymph Node Biopsy".

Entity Extraction: The doctor's order sentences retained after the above processing still have the problem of noise, so we directly extract the key medical entities in the text from the orders based on our named entity recognition algorithm. The extracted key medical entities are conceptual entities in MetaMed KE, including "organization", "disease", "observation operation", "operation", "operation method", "drug", "clinical observation", "Human body shape and structure", "orientation" and so on. Use TF-IDF to obtain high-frequency concept entities, and concatenate the filtered concept entities as the output string of this step.

4.2 Model Layer

We frame the diagnostic coding task as a multi-label classification problem. The text obtained by the preprocessing layer is concatenated and used as the model input. For the model layer, the DKPLM [16] (Decomposable Knowledge Enhanced Pre-trained Language Model) in the Chinese medical field is used as the encoder, followed by a fully connected layer to obtain the output vector. Each value of the output vector corresponds to a diagnostic coding label, then applied the Sigmoid to obtain probability. We use a threshold of 0.5 to output the labels. The loss function uses binary Focal Loss loss.

1) Pre-trained Language Model. DKPLM [16] is applied as the encoder of our model, a medical pre-trained language model using knowledge enhancement.

2) Value-Level Attention Pooling. This task is a multi-label classification problem, and there are correlations between the output labels. Only using the encoding vector corresponding to the [CLS] of the pre-trained language model to classify cannot bring enough information for multiple labels. So we proposed the Value-Level Attention Pooling (VLAP) method, considering that the output vector corresponding to each position of the input text impacts the target and decides jointly to output the multiple labels. VLAP uses the scaled-dot product attention to learn the weight of each value of each vector. It is shown in Fig. 8.

3) Label Attention and Loss. According to the data analysis, the diagnostic codes have a long-tailed distribution (label unbalanced), including 1) a large number of diagnostic codes mainly focus on tumors. 2) There are lots of candidate diagnoses in the "post-operative" time state, which is easily confused with the same type of "non-postoperative" diagnosis, such as "Course of Chemotherapy for Tumor" and "Chemotherapy for Malignant Tumor after Surgery", "Immunotherapy for Malignant Tumor" and "Immunotherapy for Malignant Tumor after Surgery". 3) The final diagnostic label may appear directly in the standardized diagnostic name, and the knowledge of anticancer drugs can play a guiding role in the diagnostic coding of cancer treatment methods, such as "Chemotherapy for Tumors", "Targeted Therapy for Malignant Tumors", etc.

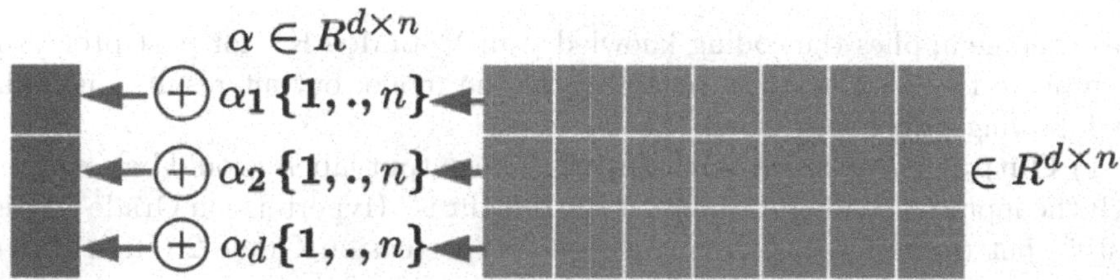

Fig. 8. Value-Level Attention Pooling

In response to the above problems, we combined knowledge and rules to design a Label Attention module to guide the network to focus on confusing and appearing in input diagnostic labels during training. We count the number of candidate diagnostic coding labels of the dataset and construct three attention vectors of the same dimension, including postoperative label attention vector v_1, prior label attention vector v_2, and label balance vector v_3. All three vectors are initialized to 0 vector, and each position of the vector represents the attention value of the corresponding diagnostic label. The calculation of the three vectors is as follows:

(1) Postoperative Label Attention Vector v_1: If the string "postoperative", the string "cancer", or terms of PNM cancer appear in the diagnostic terms before standardization, and the diagnostic terms do not contain non-target interference string, such as "intervention", "post-cesarean section", "postoperative recurrence", the postoperative treatment label for malignant tumors is considered as the candidate diagnostic label. Therefore, in the v_1 vector, assign 1.0 to the value of the corresponding position of the candidate diagnostic labels contained postoperative state, such as "Targeted Therapy after Malignant Tumor Surgery", "Immunotherapy after Malignant Tumor Surgery", etc.

(2) Prior Label Attention Vector v_2: If the diagnostic label appears in the standardized diagnostic name of the input, set 1.0 to the value of the corresponding position of the v_2.

(3) Label Balance Vector v_3: Due to the imbalanced label problem, the vector v_3 is formulated to balance the loss contribution of different labels.

v_a is calculated as follows:

$$v_a = v_1 \times (v_2 + 1) \times v_3 \tag{1}$$

In the model training stage, we use the dot-product of the v_a vector normalized by the $L2$ norm and the multi-label classification loss (using binary Focal Loss loss) as the final loss so that the optimization direction of the network tends to be emphasis-weighted diagnostic labels in v_a. The Label Attention module introduces prior label information according to the knowledge and rules to assist in training the network and improve the generalization of the network.

4.3 Postprocessing Layer

This module applies the coding knowledge in MetaMed KE for post-processing to improve the accuracy and reliability of the model output results, including the following principles:

1) Output Consistent with Input: The output labels should be consistent with the input terms. For example, if the output is "Hypertension Grade 3 (High Risk)", but the input diagnosis contains "Hypertension Grade 2 (High Risk)", the output needs to be revamped.

2) No Violation between Outputs: Diagnoses in the output label have a subordinate, a subordinate, or a sibling relationship, but they cannot exist simultaneously. As shown in Fig. 9, "Type 1 Diabetes" and "Type 2 Diabetes" will not appear in one sample at the same time, nor will "Malignant Tumor of the Upper Lobe of the Lung" and "Malignant Tumor of the Upper Lobe of the Right Lung" occur at the same time.

3) General Coding Principles: The result should be consistent with some general coding principles. For example, whether to use the code of "History of Malignant Tumor": when the diagnosed patient is in a malignant tumor, the code of history of a malignant tumor can not exist. When the malignancy is diagnosed in the past and not currently, the code of history of a malignant tumor should be used.

5 Experiments

5.1 Dataset

In the dataset of this task in CHIP2022, the input consists of admission diagnosis, preoperative diagnosis, procedure, postoperative diagnosis, discharge diagnosis, doctor's order, and drug name, and the output is ICD-10 diagnoses, using "Disease Classification and Code National Clinical Edition 2.0" as a standard diagnostic catalog. The dataset includes 2700 samples, with a total of 278 labels. We randomly divide the dataset into training, validation, and test set with a ratio of 7:1.5:1.5 and report the average performance of 5 runs from the test set.

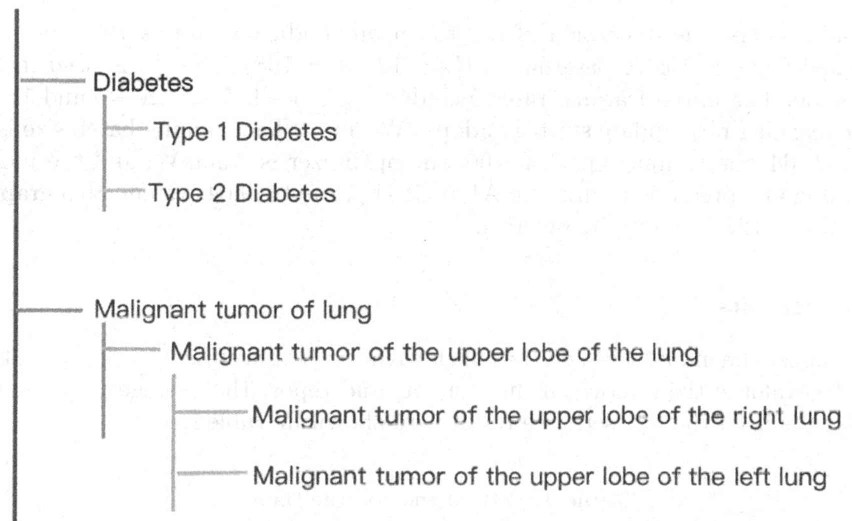

Fig. 9. Diagnosis Tree

5.2 Baselines

We compare our model with the following baselines algorithms:

(1) TFIDF+XGBoost [17]**:** Apply TFIDF to convert the text into a vector based on word frequency and input the vector to XGBoost for classification.

(2) FastText [18]**+XGBoost:** Use Fasttext to obtain the representation vector of the input text and then input it to XGBoost for classification.

(3) BERT [13]**:** We finetune BERT on the training set and then fuse finetuned BERT and other modules to represent the input text sequence for classification.

5.3 Evaluation Metrics

For this task, the common algorithm metrics are used for evaluation, including:

(1) Accuracy: The number of correctly predicted samples is divided by the total number of predicted samples. The definition of whether the prediction is correct is: if the predicted label set is entirely equal to the actual label set, it is considered correct; otherwise, it is wrong, even if the two sets have an intersection.

(2) F1-Score: The harmonic mean of precision and recall. $F1 = 2/(1/Precision + 1/Recall)$, and micro average method is used for $F1$.

5.4 Implementation Details

In all models, the dimension of the token embedding vector is 768. The pre-trained Chinese BERT-base model (L = 12, H = 768, A = 12) is used in the baseline. The initial learning rates include 2e−4, 1e−4, 5e−5, 2e−5, and 1e−5. The learning rate update strategy adopts Warmup. The training batch size is in 16, 32, 64, the training epoch is 100, the optimizer is AdamW, and the model training and prediction run on an A100 GPU (Ubuntu20.04 system, 80G graphic memory, 512G memory, 128 Cores).

5.5 Results

We choose the model saved on the epoch with the best accuracy on the validation set to evaluate the metrics on the test set, and report the average performance of 5 runs from the test set. The results are shown in Table 1.

Table 1. Performance on the Dataset

Method/Metrics	Accuracy	F1-score (micro)
FastText + XGBoost	0.0567	0.4710
TFIDF + XGBoost	0.1765	0.5887
BERT	0.3728	0.7000
BERT + Order Preprocessing	0.4025	0.7100
BERT + VLAP	0.4096	0.7203
KE + BERT + VLAP	0.4104	0.7284
KE + BERT + VLAP + Post	0.4163	0.7309
Ours (Pre + KE + DKPLM + VLAP + Post)	**0.4444**	**0.7466**

We can see from Table 1: (1) The pre-trained language model has a stronger text representation ability than traditional methods. (2) Since the doctor's order contains lots of information irrelevant to the target, the performance of preprocessing the doctor's order can be significantly improved because of the length of the text limits in BERT, resulting in important information may being truncated without preprocessing. (3) The Value-Level Attention Pooling (VLAP) we proposed can improve the performance, implying that the representation vector corresponding to each text position contributes. (4) Knowledge integration is practical, meaning that the knowledge can enhance the model in the case of insufficient samples and data. (5) In practical applications, general post-processing is necessary to alleviate the results because the model may overfit in insufficient data.

5.6 TOP15 Labels Statistics

The accuracy of our model on the TOP15 labels with the number of samples is listed in Fig. 10. The label at the bottom is not necessary for statistics because there are only a small number of samples in the test set. It can be seen that the performance of each label is related to the sample number. However, it is not wholly positively correlated, so the result of each label depends not only on the sample number but also on the distinction between labels.

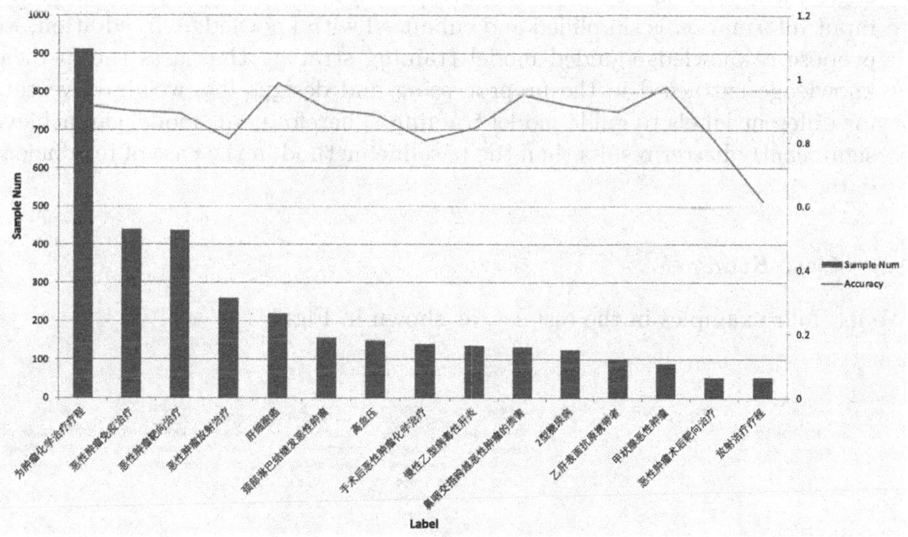

Fig. 10. TOP15 Labels Accuracy

5.7 Results Analysis

We can draw some conclusions from the results:

1) In this paper, the clinical diagnostic coding task for Chinese electronic medical records is modeled as a multi-label classification task. In the case of insufficient

data, we establish an automated clinical coding framework for Chinese electronic medical records through text preprocessing, knowledge introduction, model building, model training, and result postprocessing. This framework can improve the efficiency, accuracy, and interpretability of clinical diagnostic coding in real scenarios. In addition, unified coding knowledge and rules can be learned from the training data to avoid the defect of the subjectivity of the manual.

2) The existing clinical diagnosis coding algorithm is mainly based on ultra-short text, relying on keyword recall. It cannot directly perform clinical diagnosis coding on Chinese electronic medical records containing redundant and noisy information. We regard the clinical diagnosis coding task for Chinese electronic medical records as a multi-label classification task, which can infer hidden coding patterns according to the context information of electronic medical records. In addition, given the problems of a large number of non-standardized terms and information noise in electronic medical records, our solution designs a preprocessing module from the perspective of data quality improvement and medical knowledge integration, including term standardization, doctor's order information labeling and screening, MetaMed KE knowledge injection, and key drugs Knowledge extraction. After processing, the input information is simplified and enhanced with knowledge. In addition, we propose a knowledge-guided model training strategy that uses the medical knowledge extracted in the preprocessing and designs loss-weighted vectors for different labels to guide model training. Therefore, our model can achieve significantly better results than the baseline method in the case of insufficient data.

5.8 Case Study

We list four examples in the test set, as shown in Fig. 11.

ID	入院诊断	术前诊断	手术名称	术后诊断	出院诊断	药品名称	医嘱	真实Label	预测Label
1	右半结肠癌 肝转移术后 pt3n0m1a iva期				右半结肠癌 肝转移术后 pt3n0m1a iva期	伊立替康 双环醇 多烯磷脂酰胆碱 帕洛诺司琼 氯化钠 苯海拉明 贝伐珠单抗 阿托品 雷贝拉唑	...;二级护理; 化疗护理[嘱托];抗肿瘤化学药物配置;按肿瘤内科疾病常规护理[嘱托]; 皮下注射; 糖尿病饮食; ...	手术后恶性肿瘤化学治疗;恶性肿瘤术后靶向治疗;2型糖尿病	手术后恶性肿瘤化学治疗;恶性肿瘤术后靶向治疗;2型糖尿病
2	甲状腺功能减退症 右肺腺癌 并肺门、纵膈淋巴结 t4n3m0				甲状腺功能减退症 右肺腺癌 并肺门、纵膈淋巴结 t4n3m0		二级护理;今日结帐出院;出院小结;按放疗科常规护理;普通饮食;浅表组织彩超(套);疾病证明书;皮肤防护处理（奥克喷）;超声计算机图文报告	为肿瘤化学治疗疗程;甲状腺功能减退症	恶性肿瘤放射治疗;甲状腺功能减退症
3	食管癌 （中分化鳞状细胞癌，ct1bn0m0) 硬膜下血肿 清除术后				高血压病3级（极高危） 食管癌 ct1n0m0 硬膜下血肿 清除术后	整蛋白型肠内营养剂 水解蛋白	二级护理;今日结帐出院;出院小结 半流饮食;疾病证明书	恶性肿瘤放射治疗;高血压病3级（高危）	高血压病3级（极高危）
4	肝癌介入术后 慢性乙型病毒性肝炎	慢性乙型病毒性肝炎 肝癌介入术后	肝癌切除术+胆囊切除术	慢性乙型病毒性肝炎 肝癌介入术后	肝细胞癌 介入术后 ypcnlc iib期 慢性乙型病毒性肝炎	...;恩替卡韦;曲马多;氢氯噻嗪; 雷贝拉唑;...	...;一级护理;拟明日送or全麻下行肝肿瘤切除术[嘱托];按肝肿瘤切除术后常规护理[嘱托];按肝胆科常规护理[嘱托];...	肝细胞癌;慢性胆囊炎	肝细胞癌;慢性乙型病毒性肝炎

Fig. 11. Case Study

In the first example, there is no information related to "Type 2 Diabetes" in all the input diagnostic information. However, the string "Diabetes Diet" appears in doctor's orders, and our model can capture this key information, so the output includes "Type 2 Diabetes". Moreover, it can capture the chemotherapy drug "Irinotecan" and the targeted drug "Bevacizumab", so the output includes "Postoperative Chemotherapy for Malignant Tumors" and "Targeted Therapy for Malignant Tumors after Surgery".

In the second example, due to insufficient data, it is very difficult to determine the labels of this example. There are the item "Malignant Tumor" in the discharge diagnoses and the string "Routine Care by Radiotherapy Department" in the doctor's orders, so the output label is "Radiotherapy for Malignant Tumor", while the actual label is "Course of Chemotherapy for Tumor". It is unclear whether chemotherapy or radiotherapy was performed because the drug list is empty, possibly due to a lack of information. Generally, unless there is no mission medical service, it is impossible to have no medication when cancer patients are admitted to the hospital.

In the third example, our model classifies correctly, but there is a problem with the actual labels. The discharge diagnoses include "Hypertension Grade 3 (Very High Risk)", but the actual label was "Hypertension Grade 3 (High Risk)", which did not match the discharge diagnosis. Moreover, there is no information saying that the patient experienced radiotherapy during this visit (there is no relevant information in the doctor's order).

In the last example, the output of our model is incorrect. The procedures include the term "Cholecystectomy" and input diagnoses include the term "Chronic Hepatitis B", due to the first label is "Hepatocellular Carcinoma", then the second label should not be the label which is related to but not as severe as "Hepatocellular Carcinoma", so the second label should be "Chronic Cholecystitis".

6 Conclusions

To deal with low-quality and insufficient data problems, we design some practical preprocessing modules to simplify and mine the knowledge behind the input text, including standardization of medical terminology, extraction of key medical orders, labeling of drug usage, identification of key drugs, concept, and entity mining, etc. After preprocessing, the dataset's input is improved in quality and knowledge density.

We use the Chinese pre-trained DKPLM model enhanced by medical knowledge and Value-Level Attention Pooling (VLAP) as an encoder, followed by a fully connected layer to obtain diagnostic label classification categories. In order to maximize the use of knowledge to improve the generalization of the model, a knowledge-guided Label Attention training strategy is proposed.

In the post-processing, general coding principles are incorporated for automatic correction so that the coding of model prediction can further improve the accuracy and robustness.

Our framework automatically identifies the clinical diagnosis codes of electronic medical records. Compared with the existing algorithms, it dramatically improves the generalization and accuracy of clinical diagnosis codes. It provides an automated solution for clinical coding in the medical area. We will use it in more realistic scenarios.

References

1. The Life Science Solutions of Alibaba Cloud. www.aliyun.com/solution/healthcare/lifescience
2. ICD. www.who.int/standards/classifications/classification-of-diseases
3. Classification and Code of Diseases, GB/T 14396-2016. https://openstd.samr.gov.cn/bzgk/gb/newGbInfo?hcno=8127A7785CA677952F9DA062463CBC41
4. He, Y., Wang, C., Zhang, S., Li, N., Li, Z., Zeng, Z.: KG-MTT-BERT: knowledge graph enhanced BERT for multi-type medical text classification. arXiv preprint arXiv:2210.03970 (2022)
5. Moons, E., Khanna, A., Akkasi, A., Moens, M.-F.: A comparison of deep learning methods for ICD coding of clinical records. Appl. Sci. **15**(10), 5262 (2020). https://doi.org/10.3390/app10155262
6. Song, C., Zhang, S., Sadoughi, N., Xie, P., Xing, E.: Generalized zero-shot text classification for ICD coding. In: Proceedings of the Twenty-Ninth International Joint Conference on Artificial Intelligence, IJCAI-2020, pp. 4018–4024 (2020). https://doi.org/10.24963/ijcai.2020/556
7. Zhang, Z., Liu, J., Razavian, N.: BERT-XML: large scale automated ICD coding using BERT pretraining. In: Proceedings of the 3rd Clinical Natural Language Processing Workshop, pp. 24–34 (2020)
8. Li, F., Yu, H.: ICD coding from clinical text using multi-filter residual convolutional neural network. In: The Thirty-Fourth AAAI Conference on Artificial Intelligence (AAAI-2020), pp. 8180–8187 (2020)
9. Vu, T., Nguyen, D.Q., Nguyen, A.: A label attention model for ICD coding from clinical text. In: Proceedings of the Twenty-Ninth International Joint Conference on Artificial Intelligence, IJCAI-2020, pp. 3336–3341 (2020)
10. Cao, P., Chen, Y., Liu, K., Zhao, J., Liu, S., Chong, W.: HyperCore: hyperbolic and co-graph representation for automatic ICD coding. In: Proceedings of the 58th Annual Meeting of the Association for Computational Linguistics, ACL-2020, pp. 3105–3114 (2020)
11. Shi, H., Xie, P., Hu, Z., Zhang, M., Xing, E.P.: Towards automated ICD coding using deep learning. arXiv preprint arXiv:1711.04075 (2017)
12. Sun, Y., Liu, Z., Yang, Z., Lin, H.: Standardization of clinical terminology based on BERT. Chin. J. Inf. **4**(35), 75 (2021)
13. Devlin, J., Chang, M.-W., Lee, K., Toutanova, K.: BERT: pre-training of deep bidirectional transformers for language understanding. In: Proceedings of the 2019 Conference of the North American Chapter of the Association for Computational Linguistics: Human Language Technologies, NAACL-HLT 2019, pp. 4171–4186 (2019)
14. Brown, T., Mann, B., Ryder, N., Subbiah, M., et al.: Language models are few-shot learners. In: Advances in Neural Information Processing Systems, NeurIPS-2020, pp. 1877–1901 (2020)

15. Raffel, C., et al.: Exploring the limits of transfer learning with a unified text-to-text transformer. J. Mach. Learn. Res. **140**(21), 1–67 (2020)
16. Zhang, T., et al.: DKPLM: decomposable knowledge-enhanced pre-trained language model for natural language understanding. In: The Thirty-Sixth AAAI Conference on Artificial Intelligence, AAAI-2022, pp. 11703–11711 (2022)
17. Chen, T., Guestrin, C.: XGBoost: a scalable tree boosting system. In: Proceedings of the 22nd ACM SIGKDD International Conference on Knowledge Discovery and Data Mining, SIGKDD-2016, pp. 785–794 (2016)
18. Joulin, A., et al.: Bag of tricks for efficient text classification. arXiv preprint arXiv:1607.01759 (2016)
19. Zong, H., Lei, J., Li, Z., et al.: Overview of technology evaluation dataset for medical multimodal information extraction. J. Med. Inform. **43**(12), 2–5+22 (2022)
20. Luo, G., Kang, B., Peng, H., et al.: An overview of clinical diagnosis coding technique evaluation dataset and baseline model. J. Med. Inform. **43**(12), 10–15 (2022)
21. Luo, G., Kang, B., Peng, H., Xiong, Y., Lin, Z., Tang, B.: Overview of CHIP 2022 shared task 5: clinical diagnostic coding. In: Tang, B., et al. (eds.) CHIP 2022. CCIS, vol. 1773, pp. xx–yy. Springer, Cham (2023)

Rule-Enhanced Disease Coding Method Based on Roberta

Bo An[1,3] and Xiaodan Lv[2(✉)]

[1] The Institute of Ethnology and Anthropology, Chinese Academy of Social Sciences, Beijing, China

[2] Yuanbao Kechuang Technology Co., Ltd., Beijing, China
maybelxd@163.com

[3] Beijing Academy of Artificial Intelligence, Beijing, China

Abstract. Disease coding is crucial in medical informatics, but its complexity and sheer volume of disease codes make traditional methods ineffective. To address this challenge, this paper formulates disease coding as a classification problem, leveraging pre-trained language models and integrating domain knowledge to propose a rule-enhanced clinical coding approach. Experimental results demonstrate the effectiveness of this method, which achieved the second-best performance in the China Health Information Processing Conference (CHIP) 2022 competition.

Keywords: Clinical Diagnosis Coding · Medical Informatization · RoBERTa · Natural Language Processing

1 Introduction

Disease coding has become a critical foundation for scientific information management in medical institutions and departments. Its applications have extended to assessing medical quality and efficiency, designing clinical pathways, evaluating key disciplines, hospital accreditation, medical payment, and monitoring rational drug use. In medical practice, the assignment of disease codes based on patients' medical records is essential for managing medical case information. This process facilitates efficient and effective medical record keeping and aids in decision-making regarding patient care.

There are several disease coding schemes, but the International Classification of Diseases (ICD) [11], developed by the World Health Organization (WHO), is the most widely recognized and influential worldwide. It has become the most commonly used disease coding method globally. To suit local medical situations, China has also introduced the China's National Clinical Version 2.0 (CNCV 2.0), which has been extensively utilized in some hospitals, providing significant support for the standardization of clinical terminology and medical record coding.

Despite professional training and study, medical coders in institutions still require a significant amount of time and effort to read medical records and assign

Supported by Beijing Academy of Artificial Intelligence.

B. Tang et al. (Eds.): CHIP 2022, CCIS 1773, pp. 206–218, 2023.
https://doi.org/10.1007/978-981-99-4826-0_19

appropriate standard codes based on coding rules, as patients with various conditions undergo multiple steps in the actual consultation process, such as triage guidance, consultation, examination, follow-up consultation, and hospitalization, leading to a wide range of medical records. This process is both inefficient and expensive to learn, and the quality of the coding requires improvement, negatively affecting vital tasks such as grouping related to disease diagnosis, infectious disease reporting, and health insurance payment [1,9]. Therefore, the development of an automatic and intelligent clinical case coding method is crucial for promoting medical informatization, improving work efficiency in coding, and achieving multi-role and multi-step monitoring of coding quality.

This paper simplifies and models disease coding as a classification problem and proposes a Rule-enhanced Disease Coding method based on a Pre-trained model (RDCP). The method concatenates essential medical records with candidate disease codes, performs binary prediction using a pre-trained Roberta [4] model, and generates the final disease codes after post-processing. The method achieved an F1 score of 0.66 on the CHIP 2022 [6,7,16] evaluation clinical diagnosis coding task dataset [8], earning it the second-place ranking in the evaluation task. This outcome demonstrates the feasibility and effectiveness of the method in the disease coding task.

2 Related Work

In recent years, research has been dedicated to improving the accuracy and efficiency of medical record coding. These efforts include the application of various strategies and techniques in the field of medical informatics.

Qie et al. [2] explored the use of total quality management in enhancing the accuracy of medical insurance medical record coding. Their work demonstrated how such management practices could lead to better data quality and organization, effectively contributing to improved medical record coding outcomes.

Wang et al. [5] discussed the design and application of a medical record intelligent coding system, which utilized big data technology. This approach allowed for more advanced data processing and analysis by harnessing the power of large datasets, ultimately providing enhanced coding insights.

Lin et al. [13] analyzed the application and improvement of an automatic coding system based on electronic medical records. They highlighted the potential benefits and efficiency gains obtained by transitioning from manual to automated coding methods.

Yang et al. [12] focused on clinical term normalization using the BERT language model, enabling a more robust understanding and interpretation of complex medical jargon. By employing state-of-the-art Natural Language Processing (NLP) techniques, this research paved the way for further advancements in the automated medical record coding domain.

Zhao Qianqian et al. [15] developed an intelligent case content quality control platform to realize real-time intelligent quality monitoring for all inpatient cases at the front page, which promoted hospital's high-quality development.

Zhu Mingyuan et al. [10] based on artificial intelligence algorithms developed various models and applied them to the data of diagnosis coding as the main part of the first page of medical records, exploring the problem of ICD coding quality control under DRGs group payment mode.

Li Fuyou et al. [14] invented a method and system of surgery coding based on knowledge graph and artificial intelligence, which improved the coding quality of first pages of medical record.

Overall, these studies showcase the potential of utilizing information technology and various methodologies in significantly enhancing the accuracy and efficiency of medical record coding processes. However, continued research and development are necessary to address challenges and explore new opportunities in this evolving domain.

3 Methods

There are three steps in the proposed method. Firstly, the input dataset is preprocessed, and essential information is extracted, including the frequency and distribution of target classification codes. The actual disease codes that appear in the dataset are employed as candidate target code sets. Next, these candidate target codes are combined with the inputs and fed into a pre-trained language model-based ranking model that outputs probabilities ranging from 0 to 1 after thresholding. In the prediction stage, the model's output undergoes post-processing, such as validation, augmentation, and removal of redundant codes, before being used for final classification coding prediction. Figure 1 illustrates the system architecture of the proposed method.

3.1 Dataset and Pre-processing

Table 1 displays the sample data used in the CHIP 2022 clinical disease coding task. The data included diagnostic information for a single patient visit, such as incoming diagnosis, pre-op diagnosis, post-op diagnosis, and going-away diagnosis, as well as the name of the operation, drugs, and medical instructions. Participants were required to provide the CNCV 2.0 code for each item, and all patient visits were sourced from real medical records and tagged according to the CNCV 2.0.

To effectively classify cases in clinical settings, it is crucial to comprehensively understand each case to accurately identify the main reason for a patient. This knowledge is fundamental in coding according to the appropriate principles. It is worth noting that even cases that may appear medically similar can have vastly different codes, depending on the reason for hospitalization. This study's training data were primarily cancer-related, focusing on common diseases or virus carriers, tumors, and related treatments.

The preprocessing stage involves various approaches to process and analyze the input information from different dimensions of datasets and prediction targets, as depicted in Fig. 2. Additionally, the named entity recognition (NER) model can assist in identifying and extracting crucial clinical observations, such as diseases or surgical operations.

Diagnose. Accurate diagnosis is critical for effective disease coding. To achieve this, our proposed method leverages a named entity recognition (NER) model to extract relevant diagnostic information across multiple dimensions, including disease and other clinical observations. In addition, we apply rule-based approaches using regular expressions to identify tumor TNM staging, a crucial component of many cancer-related diagnoses.

Operation. The operative information clearly explains the reason for a patient's condition. The NER model mentioned earlier in this method extracts operations and procedures.

Table 1. CHIP 2022 Clinical Diagnosis Coding Task Dataset Sample.

Items	#Contents
Admission diagnosis	Right kidney cancer Hypertriglyceridemia Hyperuricemia Hypertension
Preoperative diagnosis	Left Right Bilateral renal tumors
Name of operation	Transabdominal right partial nephrectomy + use of artificial intelligence adjuvant therapy plus admission (si)
Postoperative diagnosis	
dischargc diagnosis	Right kidney cancer pt2an0m0 hypertension
Medicine	omega-3 fish oil fat milk alanyl glutamine lactulose diazepam celecoxib ... Recombinant human insulin r Sodium potassium magnesium calcium glucose long chain fatty milk
Doctor's advice	"3 m breathable transparent dressing (fixed catheter) 9546hp.10 * 11.5 cm. ...... To be sent to the operating room "tomorrow" for "robotic assisted laparoscopic partial right nephrectomy" under general anesthesia [self-prepared] [instructions] Routine care after robotic partial right nephrectomy under general anesthesia [self-prepared] [instructions] Change of medication (in) Change of fluids [instructions]
Target	Renal malignancy; primary hypertension

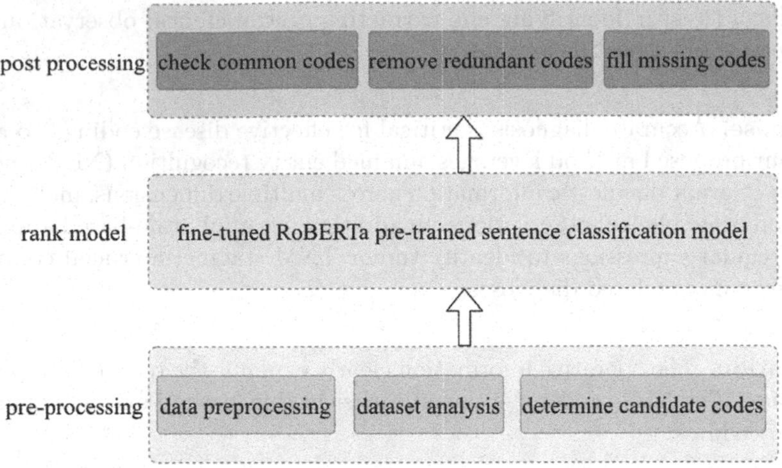

Fig. 1. The illustration of the framework.

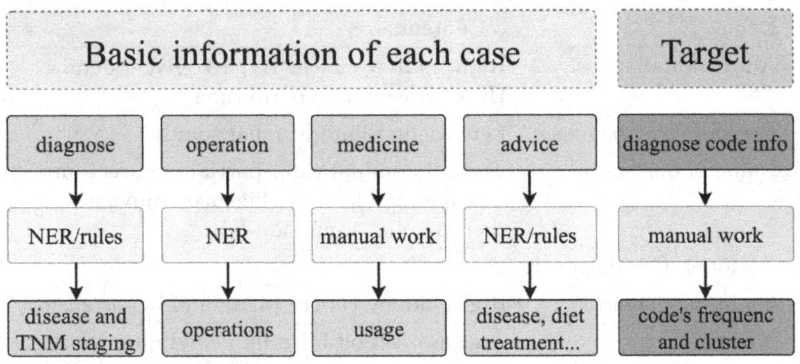

Fig. 2. Introduction of the dataset and the preprocessing step.

Medicine. The field of medicine contains information on treatments, such as chemotherapy targets, which require distinct processing from other input types. To handle drugs that appear in the dataset, medical professionals have provided summaries of their uses, particularly those related to cancer treatments.

Advice. Prescription information contains additional information that complements other dimensions, such as disease information, operation scheduling, incision size, an aesthetic level, and dietary principles. In this method, the NER model extracts the disease and operation information while rules based on relevant keywords are applied to derive the remaining information.

Target. The dataset consists of 2700 data lines labelled with codes from the CNCV 2.0 word list. This extensive list comprised over 3000 codes, some of which were closely linked and had synonyms or multiple forms in medical terminology, indicating semantic similarity. Consequently, only 278 unique codes were present in the dataset, with a significant frequency variance. These factors posed significant challenges for the classification coding prediction task.

We limited our training to the 278 disease codes in the actual task data to simplify the task. Moreover, we manually grouped frequently occurring codes into "coding clusters" based on medical knowledge and clinical expertise. Multiple codes within the same cluster were highly similar and rarely co-occurred in a standard codebook for the same diagnosis. This coding cluster information was leveraged in the post-processing stage to filter out extraneous codes.

3.2 Model Structure

In this study, we employed an approach based on the RoBERTa pre-trained model to address the problem of diagnostic coding for the medical record homepage in clinical scenarios. To achieve this goal, we added a fully connected layer and a softmax layer on top of the RoBERTa pre-trained model, thus constructing a neural network model for ranking.

The model accepts sentence pairs formed by concatenating the aforementioned pre-processed multi-dimensional information and candidate codes as input data. Moreover, by combining the multi-dimensional information with candidate codes, it ensures that the model can better understand the importance of medical record information in expressing the severity of diseases.

The model outputs a probability value ranging from 0 to 1, indicating the matching degree of the given input sentence pairs, i.e., the matching degree between the medical record input information and the candidate codes. In this way, we can obtain a set of possible diagnosis codes and their corresponding confidence levels, making it convenient for selection and judgment in subsequent applications.

Figure 3 illustrates the overall structure of the model, which consists of the RoBERTa pre-trained model, the fully connected layer, and the softmax layer responsible for generating probability values mentioned earlier. These three components together form a neural network model that effectively supports high-quality diagnostic coding for the medical record homepage.

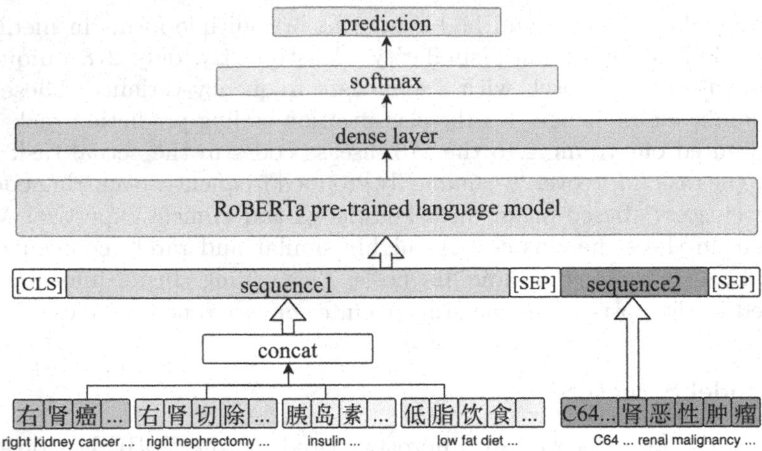

Fig. 3. The model structure.

3.3 Training Stage

In this study, we adopted a 5-fold cross-validation method to partition the dataset and train five ranking models. During the competition, we randomly selected 200 tasks for testing, while the remaining 2500 tasks were used for 5-fold cross-validation and training of the ranking model, as shown in Fig. 4. In the final prediction stage, the five models' output probabilities were averaged, pooled, and then thresholded to determine the final coding results.

In each fold of the model, as previously mentioned, only the 278 diagnostic codes that appear in the task data set are used as candidate codes for training. The ranking models rank and match these candidate codes for each input data. To preprocess the training inputs, we first partition them with [SEP] as the input for the Roberta model. Then, we take the vector corresponding to the position of [CLS] in the output of the pre-trained model as the input for the subsequent fully connected layer. This layer is followed by a softmax activation function, which transforms the problem of predicting a candidate standard code from patient information into a binary classification problem.

3.4 Prediction and Post-processing

Prediction. During the prediction stage, the probability outputs from all five models were averaged using a pooling method to determine the diagnosis code. The number of codes predicted by the models needed to be fixed and required further processing to generate the final output.

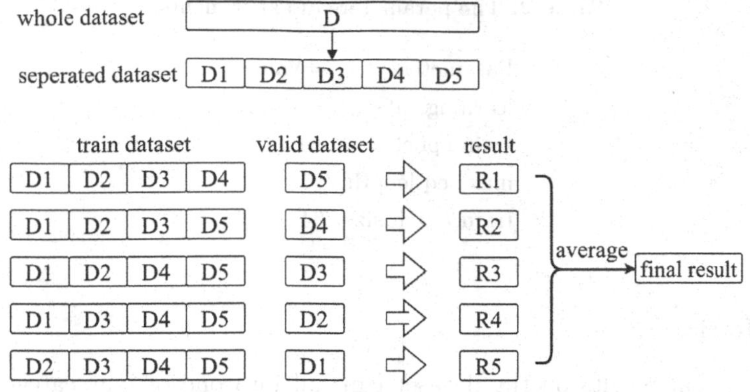

Fig. 4. The illustration of dataset partitioning and cross-validation.

Post-processing. Post-processing requires drawing on doctors' experience or medical knowledge, and incorporating it as rules into the post-processing program. This mainly includes the following steps.

Verify hypertension, diabetes, and related codes for liver, lung, and thyroid, etc. For example, if "hypertension" is clearly written in the diagnostic part of the input but the model fails to predict it successfully, "hypertension" needs to be added to the output codes.

Verify lymph node, benign and malignant, radiotherapy, and chemotherapy-related codes. For instance, verify "chemotherapy" related codes by considering chemotherapy drugs in medications.

Remove redundant predicted codes based on code cluster information. For example, normal coding results will not contain both "hypertension" and "Stage 1 hypertension" simultaneously.

Taking into account that the data for this competition comes from oncology departments, if the prediction codes do not include tumor-related information, recall and supplement important missing codes from the 30k+ codes based on medical record diagnosis information.

4 Experiments

4.1 Experimental Settings

The training set was randomly sampled from the task dataset, with a ratio of approximately 1:3 between positive and negative samples. The model was developed using the PyTorch framework and trained on an A100 GPU, with the parameters specified in Table 2.

Table 2. The parameters of experiments.

Parameters	#Value
learning_rate	2e−5
train_epoch	10
max_seq_length	512
train_batch_size	64

4.2 Metrics

The prediction results on the dataset can fall into one of four categories: (1) true positive (TP), when the model correctly predicts a positive case; (2) false positive (FP), when a negative case is incorrectly predicted as positive; (3) true negative (TN), when the model correctly predicts a negative case; and (4) false negative (FN), when a positive case is incorrectly predicted as negative.

Given a medical record with an uncertain number of standard codes, the predictions can be evaluated in either a full-correct or partial-correct manner without sorting the predictions by priors.

When evaluating predictions according to the full-correct criterion, the accuracy metric A is employed, which is defined as the proportion of cases where all diagnoses, operations, drugs, and orders in the prediction match exactly with the ground truth. When evaluating predictions based on the partial-correct criteria, the metrics are precision, recall, and F1.

We define these metrics based on the calculation of formulas. The clinical coding diagnostic task from CHIP 2022 used F1 as its final metric.

$$\begin{aligned} A &= pre\_T/N \\ P &= \frac{TP}{TP+FP} \\ R &= \frac{TP}{TP+FN} \\ F1 &= \frac{2*P*R}{P+R} \end{aligned} \tag{1}$$

4.3 Results

The model is verified on the 200 sample data divided in advance. The result is shown in Table 3.

Table 3 shows that the model's performance improves to varying degrees with an increase in the number of training epochs. The best overall result was achieved when the threshold was set between 0.3 to 0.5, with an F1 score of 46.03% for partial correct and 40.00% for full correct evaluations.

Table 3. Performance metrics at different thresholds and epochs.

Threshold	3 epoch				10 epoch			
	P/%	R/%	F1/%	A/%	P/%	R/%	F1/%	A/%
0.1	51.00	28.54	36.60	6.00	36.80	49.80	42.32	16.50
0.2	49.40	39.17	43.69	17.00	42.66	49.00	45.61	21.00
0.3	46.99	44.83	45.88	21.50	46.18	48.59	47.36	27.00
0.4	43.78	45.99	44.86	21.50	47.50	45.78	46.63	32.00
0.5	40.16	44.44	42.19	20.00	46.35	43.37	44.81	33.00
0.6	33.73	40.38	36.76	14.00	45.81	41.77	43.70	25.50
0.7	30.52	38.00	33.85	10.00	44.34	39.36	41.70	22.50
0.8	24.50	33.52	28.31	8.00	40.98	33.73	37.00	14.50
0.9	0	0	None	0	38.58	30.52	34.08	10.50

The task of disease coding requires both accurate medical knowledge and logical rules. The post-processing stage significantly improved the model's performance, as presented in Table 4.

Table 4 demonstrates that the model's performance improved as the number of training epochs increased, achieving the highest F1 score of 42.04% for partial correct and 40.00% for complete correct when the threshold was set to 0.5 epoch. Furthermore, after post-processing, the final submission of 10 epoch thresholds at 0.4 and 0.5 obtained an impressive F1 score of 66% on the official test set (which is not publicly available).

Table 4. Performance metrics at different thresholds and epochs after post-processing using rules.

Threshold	3 epoch				10 epoch			
	P/%	R/%	F1/%	A/%	P/%	R/%	F1/%	A/%
0.1	34.06	50.20	40.58	10.50	39.73	46.59	42.88	23.50
0.2	41.36	49.00	44.85	22.50	43.56	46.18	44.83	29.50
0.3	43.89	46.18	45.01	27.50	45.49	46.59	46.03	35.00
0.4	43.55	43.37	43.46	29.50	46.69	45.38	46.03	39.00
0.5	42.74	41.37	42.04	30.00	45.99	43.78	44.86	40.00
0.6	39.83	36.95	38.33	27.00	45.96	43.37	44.63	38.00
0.7	37.72	34.54	36.06	23.00	44.83	41.77	43.24	36.00
0.8	36.49	32.53	34.39	19.50	42.67	38.55	40.51	30.50
0.9	32.04	26.51	29.01	11.50	41.89	37.35	39.49	26.50

4.4 Discussions

The competition data was gathered from actual clinical records, providing a realistic depiction of the challenges and complexities of disease coding. Disease coding is an ever-evolving field, subject to shifting standards and individual coder preferences. Furthermore, the occurrence frequency of particular codes varies across different populations, making it difficult to establish universal semantic representation. Input data includes many precise medical terms that are often condensed and closely resemble one another, making them challenging too differentiate. Output labelling poses its own set of difficulties, with relationships between codes, such as synonyms, homonyms, and sub-subspecies, often indistinguishable. Moreover, each case in the data set was assigned an unspecified number of labels. The overall sample size was relatively small, and the categories were biased.

Table 5 presents an example of a "bad case" which illustrates some of the challenges of clinical coding. The table reveals that the patient was diagnosed with left breast cancer, underwent a modified radical mastectomy, and received doxorubicin chemotherapy. The cancer was classified as TNM stage pt1n2m0 (stage I), and the patient underwent radical surgery, indicating regional lymph node involvement. However, the information provided does not allow for identification of the exact quadrant where the disease occurred. Further investigation, such as examining the results of model post-processing, would be necessary to verify this information.

Table 5. Bad case.

Items	#Contents
admission diagnosis	Left breast lump
preoperative diagnosis	Invasive carcinoma of the left breast
name of operation	Modified radical surgery for left breast cancer
postoperative diagnosis	Left breast lump
discharge diagnosis	Invasive carcinoma of the left breast pt1n2m0
medicine	Medium/long chain fatty milk (c8-24) Dexamethasone Compounded amino acids (18aa-vii) Compounded licorice Dolasetron Doxorubicin liposomes Palonosetron
doctor's advice	Fasting from water and food after 8pm [instructed] Disposable oxygen inhaler ot-mi-100 type. Small size. (zero sense): 30 sets/box ... Disposable negative pressure drainage line||ay-y20-q400(f19). ... Cardiac monitoring [instructed] Removal of urinary catheter Proposed left breast cancer modified radical surgery under general anesthesia tomorrow [instructed] Preoperative care according to breast cancer routine [instructed]
target	Malignant tumor in the upper outer quadrant of the breast; secondary malignant tumor in the axillary lymph nodes; chemotherapy for malignant tumor after surgery
prediction	Axillary lymph node secondary malignancy; post-surgical malignancy chemotherapy

5 Conclusion

This paper presents a novel approach for clinical disease coding prediction using the pre-trained RoBERTa model. Our method involves converting the coding prediction task into a binary classification problem and post-processing the output to obtain the final coding result. By leveraging the power of the pre-trained RoBERTa model, our method automatically extracts critical information from the medical records and accurately predicts the correct code. Notably, in the CHIP 2022 test set, our proposed method achieved an impressive F1 score of 66%, thus demonstrating its effectiveness and feasibility in clinical coding prediction.

In our proposed method, we utilize the Chinese RoBERTa as the backbone of the model. However, it is worth exploring the potential of other medical-related BERT [3] models as a replacement in future work. Additionally, we could enhance the performance of the ranking model by incorporating more challenging negative examples. Medical knowledge plays a crucial role in addressing the disease coding problem. To leverage this knowledge, we aim to construct a knowledge graph that integrates drug and disease coding information, and fuse it with the model. This strategy can significantly improve the comprehension of medical record data and promote the generalization and performance of our method on disease coding tasks. Furthermore, it may facilitate the standardization of coding standards and quality control across various hospital levels.

Acknowledgments. This work is supported by the Natural Science Foundation of China (22BTQ010), the National Natural Science Foundation of China (62076233) and the Innovation Project major research of Chinese Academy of Social Sciences (2022MZSQN001).

References

1. Chen, F., Zhou, X., H. X.: Analysis of the influence of hospital disease automatic coding system on coding efficiency and quality. Chin. Med. Rec. **21**(11) (2021)
2. Chen, H., Chen, H., Q.M.C.L.: Application of total quality management in improving the accuracy of medical insurance medical record coding. Mil. Med. J. Southeast China **20**(1) (2018)
3. Lee, J., et al.: BioBERT: a pre-trained biomedical language representation model for biomedical text mining. Bioinformatics **36**(4), 1234–1240 (2020). https://doi.org/10.1093/bioinformatics/btz682
4. Liu, Y., et al.: RoBERTa: a robustly optimized BERT pretraining approach. arXiv preprint arXiv:1907.11692 (2019)
5. Liu, K., Zheng, L., W.Y.L.H.F.W.L.M.A.S.: Design and application of medical record intelligent coding system based on big data technology. Chin. Med. Rec. **19**(8) (2018)
6. Luo, G., Kang, B., Peng, H., Xiong, Y., Lin, Z., Tang, B.: Overview of CHIP 2022 shared task 5: clinical diagnostic coding. In: Tang, B., et al. (eds.) CHIP 2022. CCIS, vol. 1773, pp. xx–yy. Springer, Cham (2023)

7. Luo, G., Kang, B., P.H.: An overview of clinical diagnosis coding technique evaluation dataset and baseline model. J. Med. Inform. **43**(12), 10–15 (2022)
8. Luo, G., Kang, B., P.H.X.Y.T.B.: An overview of clinical diagnostic coding technology evaluation data set and baseline model. Electron. J. Clin. Med. Lit. **43**(12) (2022)
9. Min, L.: Exploration of the causes and treatment measures of disease coding errors in the front page of hospital medical records. World Latest Med. Inf. **21**(21) (2021)
10. Mingyu, Z.: Research on intelligent coding of the home page of medical records based on medical artificial intelligence technology, vol. 13 (2018)
11. World Health Organization: The ICD-10 classification of mental and behavioural disorders: clinical descriptions and diagnostic guidelines. World Health Organization, Geneva, Switzerland (2010)
12. Sun, Y., Liu, Z., Y.Z.L.H.: Clinical term normalization based on BERT. J. Chin. Inf. Process. **35**(4), 75–82 (2021)
13. Xie, L., Xiong, H., L.Z.X.F.: Application analysis and improvement of automatic coding system based on electronic medical record. Electron. J. Clin. Med. Lit. **7**(83) (2020)
14. Qin, Z., Lin, W., W.J.Y.Y.M.K.G.Q.H.N.: Study on the building and application of cancer knowledge graph for clinical decision support, vol. 42 (2021)
15. Zhao, Q., Li, L., J.Z.L.L.L.X.: Design and implementation of intelligent quality control system for the front page of inpatient medical records. Chin. Med. Rec. **23**(8) (2022)
16. Zong, H., Lei, J., L.Z.: Overview of technology evaluation dataset for medical multimodal information extraction. J. Med. Inform. **43**(12), 2–5 (2022)

Diagnosis Coding Rule-Matching Based on Characteristic Words and Dictionaries

Shuangcan Xue, Jintao Tang(✉), Shasha Li, and Ting Wang

School of Computer, National University of Defense Technology, Changsha, China
{xuescan,tangjintao,shashali,tingwang}@nudt.edu.cn

Abstract. With the continuous development of medical informatization and the wide use of electronic medical records, realizing effective informatization standard management is essential for the storage and use of medical information. The 8th China Health Information Processing Conference (CHIP2022) shared task 5 proposed diagnostic coding for Chinese electronic medical records. According to the relevant diagnosis and other seven attributes of the medical information, match its corresponding standard codings from National Clinical Version 2.0. In this evaluation task, we propose a method of matching diagnostic codings based on medical feature words and feature drug dictionaries using medical text feature words and the connection between therapeutic drugs and therapeutic means. The experimental results on the test dataset showed that the F1 value of our proposed method was 65.81%, which obtained third place in this task.

Keywords: Clinical diagnosis coding · Feature word · Rule matching

1 Introduction

In recent years, with the construction and development of medical informatization, the whole process of treatment, cost, and other information of patients in the hospital has gradually realized informatization and data. How to use computer-related technology to process massive amounts of Chinese clinical medical data is a hot issue that scholars have been studying [1]. For example, standardization of clinical terms, identification of Named Entities Recognition (NER) [2] of Chinese medical texts and Relationship Extraction (RE) [3]. Continuous mining of valuable information in medical records support medical research and decision-making of adjuvant therapy options to help doctors quickly master patient information and also improve hospital management level and efficiency to achieve better medical informatization management.

Disease classification and surgical operation classification coding is the processing of disease diagnosis and treatment information, and is an important part in medical record information management. Medical record coding has become one of the crucial bases for scientific and informatization management of hospitals. It is more and more widely used and in-depth in evaluating medical quality and medical efficiency, designing clinical pathway programs, disease

B. Tang et al. (Eds.): CHIP 2022, CCIS 1773, pp. 219–227, 2023.
https://doi.org/10.1007/978-981-99-4826-0_20

diagnosis grading, and rational drug use monitoring. In order to realize the unification of coding, the country has also launched the Disease Classification and Code National Clinical Version 2.0 and Surgical Operation Classification Code National Clinical Version 2.0. However, in the actual process of clinical records, due to the non-uniform norms related to hospitals, different professional levels, and styles of recording personnel, there are some problems such as missing important primary diagnoses or filling in the main diagnoses incorrectly.

The 8th China Health Information Processing Conference (CHIP2022) released the evaluation task of clinical diagnosis code for Chinese electronic medical records. It contains the relevant diagnostic information of a patient (including admission diagnosis, preoperative diagnosis, postoperative diagnosis, and discharge diagnosis), as well as the surgical name, drug name, medical order name, and requires to give the corresponding standard codings from National Clinical Version 2.0. The evaluation task released 2700 manually labeled medical records as training data and 337 unlabeled medical records as test data. In response to this evaluation task, we have achieved third place in the CHIP2022 clinical diagnostic coding evaluation task based on the relationship between characteristic drugs and treatment and the multi-rule diagnostic coding matching method of Chinese characteristic medical words.

2 Related Work

At present, the main methods of clinical diagnosis coding focus on machine learning methods and deep neural network-based learning methods.

Machine learning methods mainly include decision trees, SVM, and other classifiers. In 2007, the ICD-9-CM dataset was published by John et al. [4] In 2008, Farkas et al. [5] used rules to extract some short texts from electronic medical records as input and decision trees as classifiers, achieving an F1 value of 88.93% on the ICD-9-CM test set. In 2012, Kang et al. [6] optimized the conceptual normalization model based on methods such as rules and improved F1 by 12.3 to 14.1% points on the AZDC dataset. In 2014, Flat SVM and Hierarchy SVM were presented on the MIMIC2 dataset by Perotte et al. [7]. In 2015, Koopman et al. [8] extracted relevant terms from death certificates, such as CT et al. Two SVM classifiers are trained, the first to consider whether there is cancer and the second to judge the term that type of cancer. In 2016, Wang et al. [9] proposed an algorithm based on sparse regularization that uses word bag models to encode graph features and annotation features to mine and exploit disease relevance through graph structure.

In a deep neural network-based coding study of clinical diagnosis, Shi et al. [10] used RNN to code text and ICD entries separately in 2017. Then they used an attention mechanism to select a diagnostic report and compared each diagnostic description and all ICD entries, achieving an F1 value of 53.2% on the MIMIC-III dataset. In 2021, Sun et al. [11] generated the set of candidate standard words corresponding to the actual words according to the Jaccard similarity algorithm. They combined the BERT model to classify the original words, with an accuracy of 90.04% on the dataset of CHIP2019 clinical term standardized evaluation task. Based on BERT, Chong et al. [12] used the implication score and two similarity scores to reorder all candidates, with an accuracy of 94.83% on the data set of the CHIP2019 clinical terminology standardized evaluation task.

3 Task Analysis

The main objective of the CHIP2022 shared task 5 is to match diagnostic coding for Chinese electronic medical records. Given the relevant diagnostic information of a patient (including admission diagnosis, preoperative diagnosis, postoperative diagnosis and discharge diagnosis), the surgical name, drug name and medical order name, it is required to give the corresponding national clinical version 2.0 standard words. The purpose of a clinical diagnosis code is to judge the principal diagnosis and diseases by using the relevant information recorded during a visit for the patient. For example, the main diagnosis on the first page of a medical record is "卵巢癌术后" (after ovarian cancer surgery), and the surgical operation is "剖腹探查、腹腔多发肿物切除术" (exploratory laparotomy, multiple abdominal tumor resection), which is suspected of having problems. After further examination of relevant medical records, it was found that the patient had previously undergone cytoreductive surgery for malignant ovarian tumor, and was recently admitted due to multiple perihepatic and abdominal masses suggested by CT examination due to the possibility of metastatic cancer in the liver and abdominal cavity. According to the purpose of admission, surgery, and pathological results, the main disease of the patient should be "腹腔多发转移癌" (multiple abdominal metastases). As shown in the Table 1:

Table 1. A Clinical Text Data Sample

出院诊断	肝转移瘤肠型腺癌，原发灶待查
手术名称	肝肿物穿刺活检肝动脉造影+tace
术前诊断	肝恶性肿瘤肝恶性肿瘤
术后诊断	肝占位肝恶性肿瘤
入院诊断	肝恶性肿瘤
药品名称	利多卡因吡柔比星地塞米松多烯磷脂酰胆碱······
医嘱	ct/mri/pet-ct/病历带到 dsa 室[自备][嘱托] 一次性使用延长管······

According to the above seven attributes of electronic medical records, we performed a statistical analysis of the data and found some characteristics as follows:

- The seven attributes in a single medical record are not necessarily complete. There maybe some missing attributes, which are mainly manifested in preoperative diagnosis and postoperative diagnosis;

- The total number of diagnostic codings in National Clinical Version 2.0 is 37289, but there are 278 codes in the labeled data. At the same time, the number of data texts corresponding to different codings is uneven, as many as 900, as few as 4;
- Some diagnostic codings are closely related to diagnostic information, but some diagnostic codings are not dependent on diagnostic information, and more are related to some characteristic drugs;
- The contents of medical orders are generally long, and most of them focus on medical devices and use methods, which are relatively less helpful for diagnostic coding and bring some noise to clinical diagnostic coding tasks.

Based on the above analysis, we proposed a rule-matching method based on characteristic words and special drug dictionaries. Different rules are designed to realize automatic coding matching by using the discrimination of different diagnostic codings according to different characteristic words and drugs. At the same time, according to the decisive discrimination effect of special drugs on treatments and the finiteness of drugs, we establish corresponding different feature drug dictionaries for various medical treatments and then realize diagnostic codings matching.

4 Method

Figure 1 gives our proposed diagnostic coding rule-matching framework based on characteristic words and drug dictionaries, including three modules: characteristic drug dictionaries matching, characteristic words rule matching and post-processing.

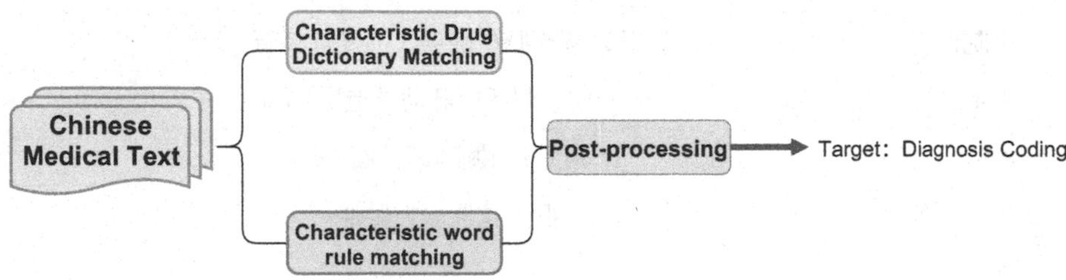

Fig. 1. The Diagnostic Coding Rule-matching Framework Based on Characteristic Words and Drug Dictionaries

4.1 Characteristic Drug Dictionary Matching

What treatment the patient receives during the hospital visit or the main diagnosis of this visit is often reflected in some drugs used for its treatment. Attributes of these drugs partly determine the matching of diagnostic codes, such as chemotherapeutic agents, targeted agents, etc. But not all drugs can be used to match diagnostic codes. Here we classify drugs into the following three categories according to their use and contribution to coding matching:

- "General drugs": some common drugs, such as glucose, sodium chloride, and so on;
- "Auxiliary drugs": drugs that play an auxiliary role in the treatment process, such as Intacted Protein Enteral Nutrition Powder;
- "Characteristic drug" refers to a characteristic drug corresponding to a certain disease or treatment, with representativeness, such as Nimotuzumab and Cisplatin.

Because of the existence of characteristic drugs, it can diagnose which type of treatment patients receive and directly match the corresponding diagnostic codings, such as "为肿瘤化学治疗疗程" (Cancer Chemotherapy Course), "恶性肿瘤免疫治疗" (Immunotherapy for malignant tumors), "恶性肿瘤靶向治疗" (Targeted therapy for malignancies), "肿瘤内分泌治疗" (Oncological endocrine therapy), "恶性肿瘤术后免疫治疗" (Postoperative immunotherapy for malignant tumors), and so on. Characteristic drugs are mainly derived from Internct-related drug website queries and drugs in the dataset. A total of four characteristic drug dictionaries were established: chemotherapeutic drugs, targeted drugs, endocrine drugs, and immunological drugs. Chemotherapy drugs contained 70 corresponding drugs, the targeted drug dictionary had 198 drugs, the endocrine drug dictionary contained seven, and the immunological drug dictionary contained 30. At the same time, the addition, deletion, and modification of the characteristic drug dictionary can also be realized according to the change in the actual situation (Fig. 2).

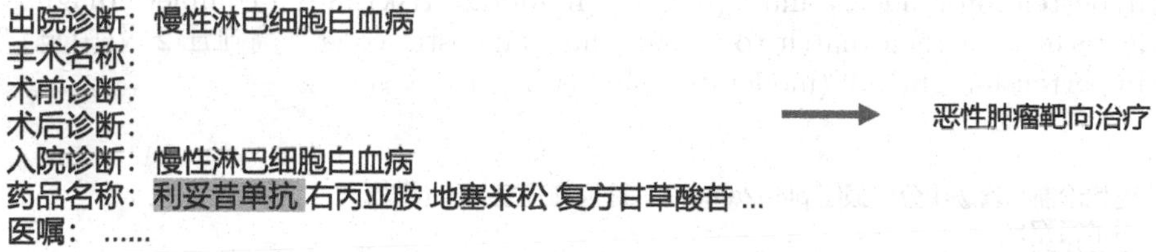

出院诊断：慢性淋巴细胞白血病
手术名称：
术前诊断：
术后诊断：
入院诊断：慢性淋巴细胞白血病
药品名称：利妥昔单抗 右丙亚胺 地塞米松 复方甘草酸苷 ...
医嘱：......
恶性肿瘤靶向治疗

Fig. 2. Example of Coding Matching Based on Characteristic Drug Dictionary. (Based on Rituximab in the drugs, we can determine the diagnostic coding is "恶性肿瘤靶向治疗" (Targeted therapy for malignancies))

According to statistical analysis, characteristic drugs appear in the medical text of drug name and medical order two attributes when the corresponding characteristic drugs are found in the corresponding text of these two attributes, and then can match the corresponding diagnostic code.

4.2 Characteristic Words Rule Matching

In terms of Chinese medical text description, it is mainly composed of general descriptions and some particular descriptions of medical treatment. These medical descriptions are mainly reflected in some characteristic words, such as "瘤" (tumor), "高血压" (hypertension), etc. These characteristic words are rare or even absent in the text description in other fields, and just represent a specific meaning in the medical field. We refer to these words collectively as characteristic words [13]. It uses the particularity and infrequence of medical text characters to realize the grading and rule matching of coding.

With as many as 278 coding types in the dataset, it is easy to cause redundancy and repetition by realizing coding matching one by one. According to the human body parts contained in the target, treatment means, and so on, we emulated the grading treatment of hospital-type objectives and divided 278 goals into 60 categories, such as lung, hypertension, breast, and so on. Each category contains different codings. For example, the hypertension category includes hypertension grade 1, grade 2, and so on. The first is to learn from the classification of hospital categories to facilitate the establishment of a rule matching function. The second is to magnify the different diagnostic codes under the same category and better mine the matching rules corresponding to the feature words or combinations.

Diagnostic information in the dataset text included discharge, preoperative, postoperative, and admission diagnosis. However, the text corresponding to the diagnosis is a long medium text string with multiple terms formed by space joins. However, we found that these terms are linked rather than entirely independent, and some terms can be merged completely to facilitate subsequent rules matching diagnostic coding. For example, for "高血压2级(中危)" (hypertension grade 2 (moderate risk)), we need to remove the space bar, combine "高血压2级" (hypertension grade 2) and "(中危)" (moderate risk) into a complete diagnostic term, and then match to obtain the diagnostic code "高血压2级(中危)" (hypertension grade 2 (moderate risk)) (Fig. 3).

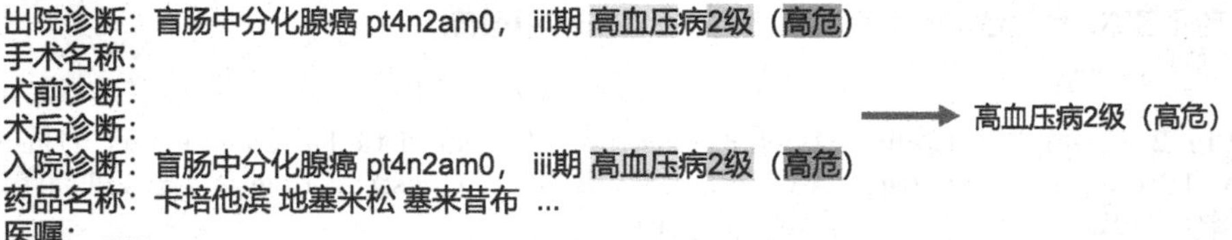

Fig. 3. Characteristic word rule encoding matching example. (We used the characteristic words: "高血压" (hypertension), "2级" (grade 2) and "高危" (high risk) to match the diagnostic coding as "高血压病2级(高危)" (hypertension grade 2 (high risk)))

In terms of characteristic words matching rules, we use diagnostic information to mine the characteristic words corresponding to diagnostic codiongs and information, as well as multiple characteristic words combinations to establish the matching rules, such as the combination of "高血压病2级(高危)" (hypertension grade 2 (high risk)) is "高血压" (hypertension), "2级" (grade 2) and "高危" (high risk). In the same coding matching process, the characteristic words combination more complex, the diagnostic coding's priority will be higher. At the same time, we also consider the compatibility between different diagnostic codings under the same kind. For example, these codings under the hypertension category are generally incompatible, but "肝囊肿" (hepatic cyst) and "乙型肝炎大三阳" (hepatitis B big three yang) under the liver category can coexist.

4.3 Post-processing

This module is mainly used to remove unreasonable and contradictory diagnostic codes and match a similar reasonable diagnostic code for coarse-graining of medical texts that do not fit the code.

Because rule matching lacks completeness and professionalism, and because of the diversity of text descriptions, contradictory and incompatible codes will appear in the actual matching process. The post-processing module needs to find these contradictory codes and retain valid codes. For example, if "乙型肝炎肝硬化" (hepatitis B cirrhosis) and "慢性乙型病毒性肝炎" (chronic viral hepatitis B) appear in the code at the same time, we will retain "慢性乙型病毒性肝炎", which is determined by our matching rules and actual coding.

At the same time, we found that there were different diagnostic codes with similar concepts when establishing the diagnostic coding rules, which we called "concept fuzzy pairs", such as "非毒性单个甲状腺结节" (non-toxic single thyroid nodule) and "非毒性多个甲状腺结节" (non-toxic multiple thyroid nodules) under the thyroid gland; such as "乳腺恶性肿瘤, 内侧" (breast malignant tumor, medial), "乳腺恶性肿瘤, 上部" (malignant breast tumor, upper), and "乳腺恶性肿瘤, 内侧" (malignant breast tumor, lateral) under the breast. These coding concepts are similar, but the difference in data text description is highly insignificant, and even manual matching of these codes has specific problems. In the post-processing, we select a similar reasonable diagnostic code as the final result.

5 Experiments and Results

5.1 Dataset

CHIP2022 Clinical Diagnostics provides 2700 manually labeled data and 337 unlabeled data, with unlabeled data as the test set. All data come from real medical scenarios.

In the next section, for better understanding, we give the micro-average precisions (P), recalls (R) and F1-scores (F1) of diagnostic codings, respectively.

$$P = \frac{TP}{TP + FP} \tag{1}$$

$$R = \frac{TP}{TP + FN} \tag{2}$$

$$F1 = \frac{2 \times P \times R}{P + R} \tag{3}$$

5.2 Experimental Results

In the paper, we use the rule-matching based on medical characteristic words and drug dictionaries to solve this task. In the experimental test, we statistically analyze the experimental results from the perspectives of medical records and diagnostic codings, which all the labeled data are used as the test set (2700 data in total). From the matching results of the entire medical record, 904 are correctly and completely matched, with a accuracy rate of 33.48%. The statistical analysis results from the perspective of diagnostic codings are shown in the Table 2.

Table 2. Testing results of our approach on the dataset released by CHIP2022.

	P (%)	R (%)	F1 (%)
Diagnostic codings	69.70	66.92	68.28

This task adopts the way of submission evaluation. The F1 value on the final official test set by using our method reached **0.6581**, which obtained the third place and proves the effectiveness of our method.

6 Conclusion

Aiming at the Chinese medical diagnosis coding task, we adopt a rule-matching method based on medical characteristic words and drug dictionaries to solve the problem of connection and matching between drug and diagnostic coding as well as diagnostic information and diagnostic coding. However, there is still room for improvement and optimization, such as the completeness and rationality of rules needing to be further improved, and at the same time, it needs to be clearly distinguished on some diagnostic codings with vague and similar concepts. Therefore, the deep network model method is reasonably added to the work to improve the method's performance further.

References

1. Huang, Y.H., Jiao, X.K., et al.: Overview of the CHIP2019 shared task track 1: normalization of Chinese clinical terminology. J. Chin. Inf. Process. (2021)
2. Li, W.X., Zhang, K.L., et al.: Overview of the CHIP2020 shared task 1: named entity recognition in Chinese merdical text. J. Chin. Inf. Process. (2022)

3. Gan, Z.F., Zan, H.Y., et al.: Overview of the CHIP2020 shared task 2: entity and relation extraction in Chinese merdical text. J. Chin. Inf. Process. (2022)
4. Pestian, J.P., Brew, C., Matykiewicz, P., et al.: A shared task involving multi-label classification of clinical free text. In: Proceedings of the Workshop on BioNLP 2007: Biological, Translational, and Clinical Language Processing. Association for Computational Linguistics (2007)
5. Szarvas, F.G.: Automatic construction of rule-based ICD-9-CM coding systems. BMC Bioinform. (2008)
6. Ning, K., Bharat, S., Zubair, A., et al.: Using rule-based natural language processing to improve disease normalization in biomedical text. J. Am. Med. Inform. Assoc. Jamia **20**(5), 876–881 (2013)
7. Perotte, A., Pivovarov, R., Natarajan, K., et al.: Diagnosis code assignment: models and evaluation metrics. J. Am. Med. Inform. Assoc. JAMIA (2014)
8. Automatic ICD-10 classification of cancers from free-text death certificates. Int. J. Med. Inform. **84**(11) (2015)
9. Wang, S., Chang, X., Li, X., et al.: Diagnosis code assignment using sparsity-based disease correlation embedding. IEEE Trans. Knowl. Data Eng. (2016)
10. Shi, H., Xie, P., Hu, Z., et al.: Towards Automated ICD Coding Using Deep Learning (2017)
11. Sun, Y.J., Liu, Z.Q., et al.: Clinical term normalization based on BERT. J. Chin. Inf. Process. (2021)
12. Chong, W.F., Li, H., et al.: Term normalization system based on BERT entailment reasoning. J. Chin. Inf. Process. (2021)
13. Xue, S., Tang, J., Li, S., Wang, T.: Hybrid granularity-based medical event extraction in Chinese electronic medical records. In: Tang, B., et al. (eds.) CHIP 2022. CCIS, vol. 1772, pp. 19–36. Springer, Singapore (2022). https://doi.org/10.1007/978-981-19-9865-2_2
14. Zong, H., Lei, J., Li, Z., et al.: Overview of technology evaluation dataset for medical multimodal information extraction. J. Med. Inform. **43**(12) (2022)
15. Luo, G., Kang, B., Peng, H., et al.: An overview of clinical diagnosis coding technique evaluation dataset and baseline model. J. Med. Inform. **43**(12), 10–15 (2022)
16. Luo, G., Kang, B., Peng, H., et al.: Overview of CHIP 2022 shared task 5: clinical diagnostic coding. In: Health Information Processing: 8th China Conference, CHIP 2022, Hangzhou, China, 21–23 October 2022, Revised Selected Papers. Springer, Singapore (2022)

3. Gan, [illegible]: Overview of the CHIP 2020 shared task 2: entity and relation extraction in Chinese medical [illegible] Inf. Process. (2022)
4. Devlin, J., [illegible] Toutanova, K.: [illegible] pre-training of [illegible] transformers for language understanding [illegible] North American Chapter of the Association for Computational Linguistics: Human Language Technologies [illegible]
5. [illegible] -based [illegible] coding system [illegible]
6. [illegible]
7. [illegible]
8. [illegible] of diseases. Int. J. [illegible]
9. [illegible] coding assignment using [illegible] based [illegible] (2010)
10. [illegible] Coding Using Deep Learning (2017)
11. [illegible] based on SGRT [illegible] (2021)
12. [illegible] (2021)
13. [illegible]
14. [illegible] (2022)
15. [illegible] (2022)
16. [illegible] Conference (2019) [illegible]

Author Index

B. Tang et al. (Eds.): CHIP 2022, CCIS 1773, pp. 229–230, 2023.
https://doi.org/10.1007/978-981-99-4826-0

Printed in the United States
by Baker & Taylor Publisher Services